BEN LOEHNEN
SENIOR EDITOR
ADULT PUBLISHING GROUP

SIMON & SCHUSTER, INC.
1230 AVENUE OF THE AMERICAS
NEW YORK, NY 10020

SIMON & SCHUSTER

September 14, 2011

Dear Reader,

If I were a doctor, or a physical trainer, or a nutritionist, or even just a good friend, I would prescribe this book. Having mastered intelligence in *The Know-It-All* and having achieved religious enlightenment in *The Year of Living Biblically*, A.J. Jacobs had one project left: bodily perfection. The result, *Drop Dead Healthy,* is not only a brilliantly entertaining book about health, but it just may be the healthiest book you could ever read.

It will make you laugh until your sides split and endorphins flood your bloodstream. It will alter the contours of your brain, imprinting you with better habits of hygiene and diet all the while infusing it with knowledge and understanding. It will move you emotionally and get you moving physically in surprising ways. And it will give you occasion to reflect on the body's many mysteries and the ultimate pursuit of health: a well-lived life.

No matter who you are—a farsighted couch potato like me or a gym-addicted Adonis like the man I resolve to be every New Year's—this book will transform the way you think about health.

Early readers here at Simon & Schuster have praised this book, and a chorus of others, including Mary Roach, Joshua Foer, Gretchen Rubin, Timothy Ferriss, and Dr. Mehmet Oz, have joined them.

You are in for a wondrous and rigorous read.

In good health,

BLoehnen
Ben Loehnen

www.simonandschuster.com
A CBS COMPANY

DROP DEAD HEALTHY

One Man's Humble Quest for Bodily Perfection

A.J. Jacobs

SIMON & SCHUSTER

New York   London   Toronto   Sydney   New Delhi

Simon & Schuster
1230 Avenue of the Americas
New York, NY 10020

Copyright © 2012 by A.J. Jacobs

All rights reserved, including the right to reproduce this book or portions thereof in any form whatsoever. For information address Simon & Schuster Subsidiary Rights Department, 1230 Avenue of the Americas, New York, NY 10020

First Simon & Schuster hardcover edition April 2012

SIMON & SCHUSTER and colophon are registered trademarks of Simon & Schuster, Inc.

For information about special discounts for bulk purchases, please contact Simon & Schuster Special Sales at 1-866-506-1949 or business@simonandschuster.com

The Simon & Schuster Speakers Bureau can bring authors to your live event. For more information or to book an event contact the Simon & Schuster Speakers Bureau at 1-866-248-3049 or visit our website at www.simonspeakers.com.

Designed by Ruth Lee-Mui

Manufactured in the United States of America

10 9 8 7 6 5 4 3 2 1

Library of Congress Cataloging-in-Publication Data

ISBN 978-1-4165-9907-4
ISBN 978-1-4391-1015-7 (ebook)

To Julie and my sons

Contents

Contents

Contents

Contents

DROP DEAD HEALTHY

Prologue

FOR THE LAST FEW MONTHS, I've been assembling a list of things I need to do to improve my health. It's an intimidatingly long list. Fifty-three pages. Here's a sample:

Eat leafy green vegetables
Do forty minutes of aerobic exercise a day
Meditate several times a week
Watch baseball (lowers blood pressure, according to one
    study)
Nap (good for the brain and heart)
Hum (prevents colds)
Win an Academy Award (A bit of a long shot, I know. But
    studies show Oscar winners live three years longer than
    non–Oscar winners.)

Keep my apartment at sixty-two degrees, since it burns more
   calories a day

Buy a potted Areca palm plant (raises oxygen levels)

Lift weights to muscle exhaustion

Become an Okinawan woman (another long shot)

And on and on.

By the way, I've printed this list in nine-point Papyrus font, because I found a study that says hard-to-read fonts improve memorization.

I want to do everything on my list because my quest isn't just to be a little bit healthier. My quest isn't to lose a couple of pounds. My quest is to turn my current self—a mushy, easily winded, moderately sickly blob—into the embodiment of health and fitness. To become as healthy as humanly possible.

I've been intrigued by the topic of health and fitness for years. But the idea of devoting myself to the cause occurred to me during a recent vacation. It was supposed to be a relaxing week with the family in the Dominican Republic. Sand castles would be built. Boggle would be played. Soda would be ordered without ice.

Instead, I ended up in a Caribbean hospital for three days with severe pneumonia. I expected some jet lag, maybe some stomach issues. But tropical pneumonia? That took me by surprise.

I'd read plenty about the importance of gratitude. So as I lay wheezing and shivering on my thin hospital mattress, I tried to find things to be thankful for. For instance, my hospital visit gave me the opportunity to learn new Spanish words such as "lung" and "pain" (*pulmón* and *dolor*, respectively). Also, roosters outside my hospital window woke me up every morning, which is marginally more charming than New York car alarms.

Neither of these observations helped much. But I found one big upside, a life-altering one. This experience was a seventy-two-hour-long memento mori. For one of the few times in my life, I was certain I was about to leave this world. Now, maybe this fear was melodramatic, but in my defense: If you were hooked up to an IV drip with a rainbow of unknown liquids (clear, yellow, blue, pink), if you saw doctors speaking in hushed tones while stealing glances at you, if you couldn't breathe without wincing, if your mind was fogged in by viruses, you might think what I did: The only way I'm getting out of here is on a stretcher covered by a sheet.

My dread was more focused than any I'd ever experienced. Probably because of my three young sons. I want to be around to see them grow up. I want to be there for their graduations, their marriages, yes, but I also want to see them sing their first Led Zeppelin karaoke song and eat their first jalapeño pepper. I want to be around to teach them the importance of having compassion and why the original *Willy Wonka* is superior to the remake. I worked myself into quite a state by imagining all of the memories I'd never have.

The thing is, I'm forty-one. I can no longer take my health for granted. Catching pneumonia is just one sign that I'm deteriorating. My bones are becoming lighter and more porous. My muscles are shriveling. My brain is shrinking, my arteries narrowing, my coordination slowing. I'm losing 1 percent of my testosterone a year.

And I'm fat. Not morbidly obese. I'm what's described as skinny fat. A python-that-swallowed-a-goat type of body. Which I've learned is the worst kind of fat. So-called visceral fat (which surrounds the liver and other vital organs) is considered much more dangerous than subcutaneous fat (the kind under the skin that causes cellulite). In fact, the size of your waistline is one of the best predictors of heart disease.

My wife, Julie, has been nudging me for years about my growing belly. She's got a repertoire. She'll refer to me as Buddha. Or she'll ask, "So, when are you due?" When she wants to be especially subtle, she'll just whistle the *Winnie-the-Pooh* theme song as she walks by.

She tells me she doesn't care about whether or not I look fat. She says she just wants me to take care of myself so I'm around. A couple of years ago, she sat me down at the dinner table, put her hands on mine, looked me in the eyes, and told me: "I don't want to be a widow at forty-five."

"I understand," I replied solemnly. I pledged to join a gym, and at the time, I meant it. But inertia is a powerful force.

So I did nothing. I continued eating food loaded with empty calories—lots of pasta and corn-syrupy cereal. There was a notable lack of anything green, not counting bottles of Rolling Rock. My exercise regimen was just as bad. I hadn't done serious aerobic exercise since college. I got winded playing hide-and-seek with my sons.

And then I found myself in the hospital gasping for air. And so, right about when the nurse came into my room bearing a pill the size of a bottle cap, I made a pledge: If I make it out alive, my next project will be about revamping my body.

I say "next project" because this book isn't my first foray into radical self-improvement. Over the last decade, I've had a bit of a fixation. Studies show it's healthy to have a purpose in life, and mine has been a relentless, well-intentioned, if often misguided quest for perfection. Project Health will be the third leg of a triathlon devoted to upgrading my mind, my spirit, and my body.

Some quick context: The mind was first. After college, away from research papers and seminars, I worried my brain was slowly turning to the consistency of Greek yogurt (which is on my list of foods to eat, incidentally). I could feel my IQ gently ebbing away. So I came up with a fix: I pledged to read the entire *Encyclopedia Britannica* and learn everything I could. It was an extreme measure, sure, but not without family precedent. I got the idea for this quest from my father, who had started to read our *Britannica* set when I was a kid, but only made it up to the letter *B*, around "Borneo" or "boomerang." I wanted to finish what he began and remove that black mark from our family history.

The alphabetical journey—which I chronicled in my first book—was painful at times. Including for those around me (my wife started to fine me one dollar for every irrelevant fact I inserted into conversation). And frankly, I've forgotten 98 percent of what I'd learned. But it was also an amazing experience. Uplifting even. After eighteen months of reading about the sweep of history, I emerged with more faith in humanity. I read about all the unfathomably evil things we've done, but also all the mind-boggling good ones (the art, the medicine, the flying buttresses of Gothic cathedrals). On balance, it seemed the good outweighed the bad, if only by a sliver.

Having checked off the mind, I was inspired enough to work on my spirit. I chose this next because I grew up without any religion or spirituality at all. As I wrote in a book on this project, I'm Jewish, but I'm Jewish in the same way the Olive Garden is Italian. Not very. But my wife had just given birth to our first son, and we were grappling with what to teach him about our heritage. So I decided to learn the Bible inside out—by living it.

I chose to follow all of the Good Book's hundreds of rules. I wanted to obey the famous decrees, like "love thy neighbor" and the Ten Commandments. But I also wanted to pay attention to the often-ignored, lesser-known rules, such as "don't shave your beard" "don't wear clothes of mixed fibers." I wanted to see which would improve my life and which were not so relevant to twenty-first-century America.

It was another experience that was simultaneously profound and absurd, manufactured and life-changing. When the year ended, I shaved my Ted Kaczynski–like facial hair and started wearing poly-cotton blends again, but I've kept much from my biblical life. I try to observe the Sabbath for instance, and to be grateful, and to avoid gossiping. "Try" is the key word here, especially on the gossip one.

Which brings me to the final quest, the last leg of the bar stool: Remake my body.

As with my other adventures, this one is fueled, in good part, by ignorance. I know astoundingly little about my own body. I know the small intestine comes before the large intestine. I know the heart is the size of a fist and that it has four chambers. But the Krebs cycle? The thymus? Presumably I read about them in the encyclopedia, but they are not in the 2 percent I retained.

And even more to the point, I don't know what to eat or drink or the best way to exercise. It's a bizarre situation. It's like owning a house for forty-one years and being unaware of the most basic information, such as how to work the kitchen sink. Or where to find the kitchen sink. Or what this so-called kitchen is.

I see this project as a crash course in my own body. I'll be a student of the strange land inside my skin. I'll try out diets and exercise regimens. I'll test drugs and supplements and tight-fitting clothes. I'll experiment with the most extreme health advice, because, as I learned in my year of living biblically, only by exploring the limits can you find the perfect middle ground.

At the end of the project, I probably won't keep up all my healthy behaviors, but I'll keep a bunch. I'll find the ones that work best. And that, I hope, will keep me alive long enough to teach my kids how to be healthy.

The Warm-Up

As with any physical endeavor, you need to warm up. You can't just start doing squats and eating kale without knowing what's what.

First thing I did was to assemble a board of medical advisers. I don't have an M.D. after my name, but—through luck and persistence—I've gotten access to the best health minds in the country. It's a somewhat ad hoc group, but varied and esteemed and far more knowledgeable than I.

I'll be getting advice from Harvard professors and Johns Hopkins researchers, from top-of-their-field doctors and from fitness trainers with biceps like cantaloupes. My aunt Marti will weigh in. She is the single most health-minded person in America, and has a mail-order business that sells powdered blue-green algae supplements and organic hand sanitizers. She lives in Berkeley and will be giving me a distinctly Californian point of view.

When I called her to tell her about the project, she was thrilled at first, then appalled. "You're doing a project on health and you're calling me from your *cell phone?*" She went on to lecture me on its brain-frying dangers. And for calling too late, since staying up at night disrupts my circadian rhythm.

I've been devouring health books and magazines and blogs. I've read at least fourteen articles on the benefits of blueberries. I'm stepped in my omega-3s and flavanoids. I know a lat from a delt, fructose from sucrose, HDL from LDL. I know that you should eat a lot of the Indian spice turmeric, as it fights cancer. Also that you should avoid the Indian spice turmeric, as it might contain dangerous levels of lead.

The research so far has been fascinating, often confusing—but overall heartening. Admittedly, I'm saddled with twenty-three pairs of chromosomes I can't change, at least not yet. But there's so much I *can* control. An estimated 50 percent of our health is determined by behavior. Our well-being is an accumulation of hundreds of little choices we make every day—what to eat, drink, breathe, wear, think, say, watch, and lift.

My timing is lucky as well. This is a good era in which to pursue total health. We've had more medical advances in the last thirty years than, arguably, the last millennium.

But I also have to be careful. I've spotted an astonishing amount of what even I—with my currently limited expertise—can tell is quackery. You'd think that with the steady march of science, the dubious health advice would have faded since the days of "Dr. Hammond's Nerve Medicine and Opium Blend." Not so.

Thanks to the Internet, just about any quarter-baked idea ever conceived still gets traction. Case in point: trepanning, a practice that dates back to 6500 BCE and involves drilling a hole in the skull to let out evil spirits.

So I did an Internet search. And guess what? It's still around. Check out the International Trepanation Advocacy Group. Its website features images of green-tinted brain scans next to doctors in white lab coats writing complicated math equations on boards. Apparently, this is not your caveman's trepanation. No, this is totally scientifical drilling of holes in your skull.

Now, quackery can be interesting and even important. (For instance, one of the leaders of the 1773 Boston Tea Party riled up the protesters by claiming that tea was hazardous to the health; so our very country is founded on absurd medical claims.)

But I want this project to be an evidence-based makeover. I want to separate the hard science from the squishy claims. I've got to be wary of the Latest Study Syndrome. Our brains are unduly drawn to whatever yesterday's study revealed—*Look at that! Bacon IS healthy*—especially if the conclusion is surprising and counterintuitive and delicious. Each study needs to be weighed against the mountain of existing data. I want to focus on the meta-analyses. Or better yet, meta-analyses of meta-analyses. I'll be seeking second opinions, but also third, fourth, and eighth opinions. I'll be consulting the Cochrane Collaboration, which sounds like a shady international conspiracy but is actually a nonpartisan group that reviews medical studies.

The trick, though, is to avoid quackery at the same time as maintaining childlike enthusiasm for innovation. Because cutting-edge medical science veers into the surreal. It's a world where mice live twice as long when they're on the verge of starvation, and where placebo inhalers for asthma improve lung performance.

I read a quote from Carl Sagan that I printed out and put on the wall above my computer. It will be my guide:

> What is called for is an exquisite balance between two conflicting needs: the most skeptical scrutiny of all hypotheses that are served up to us and at the same time a great openness to new ideas.

The Battle Plan

What does it mean to be maximally healthy? Courtesy of the World Health Organization's definition of health, I've broken it down to three parts:

1. Longevity
2. Freedom from disease and pain
3. A sense of emotional, mental, and physical well-being

If I can have those three, I'll be ecstatic. It'd be nice to get a six-pack, but it's not my top priority—unless I decide I need shredded abs for emotional well-being, as many magazines seem to imply.

I'm going to quantify my progress as best I can. Granted, the longevity part will be tough to measure, unless I happen to die during my project. Which would be embarrassing, but would certainly provide some closure. But the other two, thankfully, are testable.

To quantify how badly off I am at the start, I visited a clinic in Rockefeller Center called EHE, short for Executive Health Enterprises.

The website boasts of the company's illustrious history: EHE has been doing preventive medicine since 1913. The founding chairman of its board? Former president William Howard Taft. Which frankly isn't the first name that comes to mind when you think of healthy living. This is a man who got stuck in the White House bathtub and had to be lifted out by four government employees.

But still, EHE is a classy joint filled with reputable doctors, and fancy clientele from law firms and banks. They offer a top-to-bottom physical and a full report card on your body. I went one morning, and it took three hours and involved six vials of blood, forty-two tests, six nurses, and eleven horrific minutes on a treadmill.

Here's what they found:

Height: 5'11". Weight: 176 pounds. Body fat percentage: 18. Total cholesterol: 134 (it used to be over 200, but I've been taking Lipitor for three years). I'm myopic. I have abnormally low hematocrit, which means the percentage of red blood cells is depressed, which could explain my fatigue. I have a heart murmur and elevated liver enzymes.

Far from perfect, but not terrible. Overall, I should be grateful I don't have any debilitating diseases. Just the usual American sloth-related maladies.

Though I should mention this was just the first test. In the coming months, I will submit myself to dozens of additional exams and find out an alarming number of other things wrong with me. Among them: sleep apnea, depleted iron, deviated septum, collapsed nostril, precancerous skin growths, and, particularly embarrassing for someone who works at a men's magazine: low testosterone. But I'm getting ahead of myself.

As my start date approached, I realized just how overwhelming being maximally healthy is. It will consume my every waking hour, and my sleeping ones, too.

I need some structure. Taking a cue from the digestive system, I've decided to break my project down into smaller, bite-size chunks. I will improve my body one part at a time. I will attempt to have the healthiest heart and the healthiest brain. But also the healthiest skin, ears, nose, feet, hands, glands, genitals, and lungs.

I know all the body parts are all linked on some level. But I want to lavish some individual attention on each.

And where to start? Since diet is such a huge part of health, I've chosen the stomach as my jumping-off point. The first part will be about what to put in my Buddha-like belly.

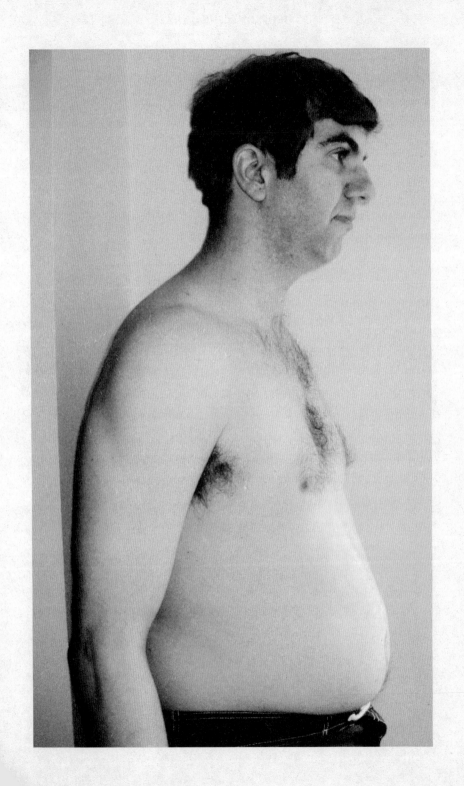

Chapter 1

The Stomach

The Quest to Eat Right

I'VE MADE A LIST of more than a hundred diets. The Mediterranean diet. The USDA diet. The Michael Pollan eat-what-your-grandparents-ate diet. The Blood-type diet. The Paleo diet. The Okinawa diet. Veganism. Raw foodism. Not to mention the more outré ones, like The Cookie Diet. The Rastafarian diet. The Master-Cleanse diet.

I want to try them all. Well, maybe not the Taco Bell Drive-Thru Diet. But most of the others. Eventually, that is. The thing is, studies show that if you switch habits too rapidly, the changes don't stick. So my plan is to wade into my new diets slowly, like my five-year-old son entering a chilly pool.

Which is how I've decided on my first dietary reforms: more chocolate, booze, and coffee.

"*Salud*," I say to Julie as I pour a cup of Starbucks Gold Coast on my first morning.

That night, our friends Paul and Lisa—who are visiting New York from D.C.—come over for an informal Thai dinner. Before the meal, as we wait for the delivery guy, I hand out glasses of Pinot Noir, and dig out a Toblerone bar from the fridge.

"So when does your health thing start?" Paul asks.

"It started today," I say, breaking off a triangular chunk.

Paul gives me a questioning look.

"He also had two cups of coffee this morning," says Julie. "That's his new health plan: chocolate, coffee, and wine."

"All very good for you," I say.

"Huh. Sounds like you're really committing yourself to this project," says Paul.

"How about heroin?" asks Lisa. "I hear that it's loaded with antioxidants."

Everyone has a good laugh.

Clever. But the science is on my side. Consider:

- Studies show that moderate drinkers live longer than both teetotalers and heavy drinkers. For men, one to two glasses a night lowers the risk of heart disease. For women, one glass is recommended. Red wine also has beneficial chemicals like resveratrol, which might have age-resistant properties.
- Dark chocolate is, in fact, loaded with antioxidants and has been shown to cut the risk of heart disease. It's also might be good for the eyes. According to one study, chocolate improves contrast sensitivity.
- Coffee lowers the odds of several types of cancer (bladder, breast, prostate, and liver) as well as Alzheimer's. It has

some downsides (more than two cups can cause sleeplessness and raise cholesterol), and isn't quite as healthy as its cousin green tea, but drunk in moderation, coffee's benefits outweigh the risks.

Still, I do understand Paul and Lisa's skepticism. In general, food that tastes good is bad for the body. As Jack LaLanne liked to say: "If it tastes good, spit it out."

Which is a bizarre situation. Evolution has betrayed us here. The human body—as miraculous as it can be—is in many ways a malfunctioning machine, a biological version of a 1978 Ford Pinto.

If evolution worked perfectly, healthy food would taste delicious and unhealthy food would make us gag. On Halloween, kids would fill their pails with quinoa and cauliflower. McDonald's would sell billions of bok choy burgers.

The problem is, we live in a modern world, but we're stuck with caveman taste buds. When our ancestors roamed the plains, our preferences actually did make sense: Our tastes aligned with healthy foods. We evolved to like sugar because it's in fruit. And fruit—which is rare in the wild—is high in nutrients, fiber, and calories. We evolved to like salt, because the body needs salt to retain water. Salt—also rare in the wild—was an occasional lifesaving treat.

But then we figured out how to extract sugar from plants and put it in pastries and Frappuccinos. We mined salt and stuck it in our soups and burritos and neon-orange cheese snacks. And in large quantities, sugar and salt are not so good for you at all.

We also started to live longer. We cured a lot of infectious diseases, but this presented a new problem. Foods that were healthy in the short run—like those loaded with fat to allow the caveman to survive the famine until the next kill—turned out to be damaging in the long run.

My question is, can I reprogram myself to love healthy food? And can I figure out how to prepare and buy healthy food that doesn't taste like a roll of double-ply Bounty?

The answer, it turns out, is yes. Sort of. But not yet.

Right now I'm still comforting myself with my holy trinity of chocolate, coffee, and booze—three of the rare foods that are already both tasty and healthy.

At least somewhat healthy. The more I research, the more I realize the situation is complicated. Consider chocolate. What's really healthy is the 100 percent cacao chocolate. No sugar, no butter.

I click onto rawcacao.com and order a bag. The mouthwatering write-up says it's "certified organic, raw, low fermentation, non-fumigated, fair traded, strict farming standards, training and equipment provided, fair wages, profit reinvestment plan, purity testing."

My bag of certified-organic-raw-low-fermentation-etc. chocolate arrives three days later. I take a pinch of the sprinkle-size nibs and pop it in my mouth. I can taste the chocolate I know from Hershey's Kisses, but it's faint and muffled, like a clock radio stuffed under a heap of pillows. Mostly I taste the bitterness.

"What's that?" Julie asks, walking into the kitchen for a snack.

"Natural chocolate," I say.

Reflexively, I offer her the bag. She takes a handful and puts it in her mouth.

I probably should have mentioned the tastes-like-chalk part, but, well, it happened so fast. Also I was curious to see her reaction.

A second. Two seconds. There it is: the same face she made when our friend showed us an Internet video of two women violating several cultural and hygienic taboos.

Taming The Portion

In my quest for healthy eating, I know I'll have to do better than my Vice Diet. But I still haven't committed to veganism or Atkins yet. I'm still too overwhelmed by choices.

I do, however, notice that there's one thing almost every nutritionist agrees on: We eat too much damn food.

We have a size problem. You can see it in the puberty-like growth spurt of portion sizes. In 1916, a bottle of Coca-Cola was 6.5 ounces. Today, it's 20 ounces. A hamburger used to be about 300 calories. Now you can enjoy Hardees' Monster Thickburger with 1,420 calories, not counting fries. (The average man should eat about 2,500 calories *a day.*)

So I've decided to split up my food reforms. First, I'll deal with quantity. Then I'll take on quality.

How to eat less? One idea is to suppress my appetite. I've read reputable studies saying a glass of water before a meal reduces the average number of calories people consume. Same goes for cayenne peppers. And an apple. And a handful of walnuts. So that's my breakfast this morning: cayenne peppers, water, an apple, and walnuts.

I won't be hungry for days! Or at least until 10 a.m. when I get the urge to snack again.

I'm going to need some professional help. Which is why, on a Sunday afternoon, Julie and I drive to a house in Westchester.

I'm here to meet the leaders of the Calorie Restriction movement. You might have heard of CR, as it's called. It's the most extreme diet you can find that isn't technically a psychological disorder or human rights violation.

The idea is that if you live on the edge of starvation, you will increase your life span. If you can survive on 30 percent fewer calories a day—say 1,750 instead of the usual 2,500 for an adult male—you'll slow down your metabolism and be free of disease. You can easily break the century mark, maybe even the 120 mark or more.

It's not an insane notion. Actually, there's a good amount of scientific data behind it, going back to a Cornell University study in 1934. Researchers were able to double the life span of mice when they fed them extremely low-calorie diets. Similar results have been found for worms, spiders, and monkeys.

Scientists still aren't 100 percent certain why calorie restriction lengthens animal life spans. One theory is that the famished animals produce fewer cell-damaging free radicals. Another says that their bodies sense starvation and switch into a defensive state, slowing their metabolism.

Does it work on humans? Studies are under way, but it's too soon to tell. The prospect, though, has attracted thousands of Calorie Restrictors, folks who weigh their food on digital scales, plot precious calories on spreadsheets, eat two meals a day, and treat their mouths like an exclusive SoHo VIP club where only the most deserving morsels can enter.

The house is perched on a steep hill atop a series of perilous turns that leave Julie frazzled. "If they want to live forever, they might want to move to a safer street," she says. Julie drops me off, and drives away to visit some friends nearby. She says I can fill her in later.

A man answers the door. He's Paul McGlothin, the director of research for the nonprofit Calorie Restriction Society, and coauthor of the how-to book *The CR Way*.

He's skinny, but not the POW skinny I was expecting. More like lead-singer-of-an-emo-band skinny.

"Welcome," he says. "Would you like some tea?"

I agree to some naturally low-calorie dandelion tea. We're in a room with minimal decorations and a huge window overlooking a forest of oaks. An event organizer by day, Paul is slope-shouldered, but sprightly for a man of sixty-four years. He's got piercing green eyes, a deep voice with a little twang from his native Tennessee, and is partial to wearing tracksuits.

We sit at the table with his wife and coauthor, Meredith Averill, sipping our tea.

"The goal of calorie restriction is not to lose weight. It's to be as mentally and physically healthy as possible. But you will lose weight." Paul went from 163 pounds to 136.

Paul eats a big breakfast (e.g., salmon, barley, lots of vegetable soup), a smaller lunch (e.g., veggie smoothie, veggie spread and sprouted grain bread)—and no dinner.

I have to restrain myself from making the same joke I know they've heard a thousand times. Yes, maybe you'll live longer, but without lasagna and pastries, who the hell wants to? (Or the alternate: You may not live longer, but you'll sure *feel* like you've lived a century and a half.)

Paul shuts down that cynical line of questioning before I get to it. He loves his gorge-free life. Loves it. "I literally get high from it," he says. "Calorie restriction makes me feel better in every way— physically and mentally."

His hand is resting on his chin, the wrist at a sharp ninety-degree angle. I can see a road map of blue veins in his arm.

Among other things, says Paul, the diet clears him of brain fog—he competes in chess tournaments against people half his age. "I played this one guy—a grand master—who was overweight and scarfed down three pizzas. I knew if I could just hold on, his body would crash. So that's what I did."

But I'm still puzzled how can they sustain the diet in a world that is so food-centric. Humans organize our very lives around meals.

"There's such an unbelievable myth that eating a lot is a way to have fun," says Meredith. "But of course, it isn't. When you're around CR people, they're usually quite active and elated."

Paul jumps in: On Christmas and Thanksgiving, he likes to fast instead of feast. No eggnog necessary: "If you're on CR, you're kind of high because you're feeling good in the first place. You feel like interacting with people and that brings out great conversations."

When you're doing CR, you have to make every bite count. Which is why Paul came up with something called "savoring meditation." I had read about the practice in his book, and ask if we could try it out.

Paul obliges, and gets a bowl of blueberries from the fridge.

We close our eyes and breathe in and out for a few minutes, like "leaves blowing in a wind." Then he starts.

"And can you imagine in your mind's eye that someone has left you a gift."

Paul speaks soothingly, in a Mr. Rogers–ish tone.

"And that gift is going to nurture you and your body in very special ways. And as you enjoy breathing in and out, you're coming to know that gift is a blueberry. Can you imagine reaching into a bowl and taking just one blueberry, just one, and putting it up to your lips. You begin to smell what that blueberry smells like. And how does it smell? Would it be musty?

"And so in your mind's eye, you take that blueberry and put it into your mouth . . . and imagine how it might get from your lips to your teeth. And without biting into it, just have it there on the tip of the tongue . . ."

By this time, Paul has me salivating. He's a tongue-tease.

"Could you taste it on the back of the tongue? On the roof of

your mouth? Can you let the taste sensation permeate your entire brain, your entire mouth, your nose?"

I. Want. That. Blueberry.

"And now, can you actually put one blueberry into your mouth in slow motion, just like they do on those instant-replay cameras in sports. And hold it there without biting it. And your brain and your tongue and the roof of your mouth and your cheeks are all participating in the experience. And when you're ready, can you begin to bite into it? Just very slowly. Can you taste the very subtle skin of the blueberry and how it meshes with the fleshy inside?"

Oh man, can I.

It went on like that for several minutes. I tell you, a blueberry never tasted so good. It's an odd and goofy ritual, if not bonkers, but if you can't appreciate a blueberry after doing twenty minutes of savoring meditation, you have a tongue made of stone.

I leave Paul's house with this lesson: I need to be mindful of what I eat. Maybe I don't need to spend fifteen minutes contemplating a blueberry. But focusing on what I put in my mouth is a key to health. As Cornell psychology professor Brian Wansink points out in his book *Mindless Eating*, one of the major causes of the obesity epidemic is that we thoughtlessly shove omnipresent food into always-open maws.

We love to multitask while eating, a sure way to get fat. Studies show that we eat up to 71 percent more when we're watching TV. (And that the number also varies depending on what we're watching; one study showed that subjects who watched *Letterman* ate more than those who watched *Leno*, which seems a good marketing opportunity for NBC. We eat more when we eat while driving, and working, and walking.

I know whom to blame for this epidemic, incidentally. When I read the encyclopedia, I learned about the father of distracted eating. He was an eighteenth-century British gambling addict who invented a food he could snack on without interrupting his card game. His name was John Montagu, the Fourth Earl of Sandwich. So the humble sandwich, much as I love it, has caused a whole lot of trouble.

The Most Mindful Eater in the World

I get home, determined to be the most conscious and aware eater in America. That went to hell the next day.

I was busy with an article for *Esquire* magazine—where I work as a writer—and at about 11 a.m., I noticed an empty plastic container and spoon on my desk. Somehow, I had managed to consume an entire cup of syrupy peach slices. It wasn't me, actually. It was some semisentient, high-fructose-loving, zombified version of me.

I need help. What I need to do is treat myself like a lab rat. I need to work from the outside in. I need to change my food environment. I call up several behavioral scientists—including Sam Sommers at Tufts University, who wrote a book called *Situations Matter*—to figure out how to design a fat-fighting apartment.

On Wednesday night, I invite—or force—the family to join me for a special dinner. It's my wife and I, and our three sons—Jasper, who is five, and his twin brothers, Lucas and Zane, who are three.

"That's quite a setup you have there," Julie says.

"Thank you."

My place setting consists of:

- My son's plastic dinosaur plate, since it's only nine inches across. (We tend to eat whatever's on our plate, so smaller plates means fewer calories.)

- A cocktail shrimp fork, since that will make me eat slower than if I had a big fork. (The slower we eat, the less total food we stuff in. This is because the body, God bless it, is dumb and slow. It takes twenty minutes for the "I'm full" message to go from the stomach to the brain.)
- A small makeup mirror propped up by my place mat. (Studies show you eat less if you watch yourself doing it.)

Tonight's dinner is whole-wheat pasta with tomato sauce and carrots. I've plated my food in the kitchen so as not to have extra on the table, tempting me.

We're not a religious family. We don't say grace. But I want my kids to realize the food didn't spontaneously generate on their plates.

"Should we talk about where this food comes from?" I ask.

"The grocery store," says Jasper.

"Well, yes. But even before that, someone had to grow the tomatoes. And someone had to pick them. Someone else had to put them in a box, and someone had to drive them in a truck. So we should appreciate how much it takes to get food on the table."

My sons pause.

"And after we eat it, it will go in the toilet," Jasper says.

For the five-and-under set, this is a bon mot worthy of George S. Kaufman. They are off and laughing.

"And after it's in the toilet, it goes into the ocean," adds Zane.

I'm still amazed at my sons' ability to turn any topic—not just food, but airplanes, LEGOs, Australia—into scatology. I guess it's better than nothing. Food mindfulness doesn't have to stop in the stomach.

I take a bite and chew. And chew some more. I've been reading these pro-chewing websites on the Internet. It's a surprisingly passionate movement. One member calls it "chewdaism." They quote Gandhi ("chew your drink and drink your food") and pro-chewing poems ("nature will castigate those who don't masticate"). They sell chewing aids, such as a CD that chimes every minute, directing you to swallow. They revere the grandfather of the pro-chewing movement, a nineteenth-century health guru named Horace Fletcher, who counted John D. Rockefeller and Kafka among his followers. They say chewing will cure stomachaches, improve energy, clear the mind, cut down on gas, and strengthen the bones.

Those claims are overblown. But chewing does offer two advantages: You can wring more nutrition out of your food. And more important, chewing makes you thinner, as it forces you to eat more slowly.

Julie wants to ask me something, but I keep my finger in the hold-that-thought position. I chew thirty times, until my noodles are so liquid they slide down my throat.

After fifteen minutes, the kids have abandoned the table. Julie is in the other room checking her e-mail. But I'm still here, alone, chewing my food and watching myself in the mirror. Slow food and children under six—that's a tricky combination. Something to work on.

Eating For Longevity

Maybe I'll have better luck with a meal with my grandfather. He's ninety-four, so I figure perhaps he's got more patience. And better yet, I can learn a thing or two from him about longevity.

He lives in a small apartment on Sixty-first Street, where I have visited him every couple of weeks for the last ten years. I open the door, and find him in front of his huge computer screen, glasses perched on the tip of his nose, tapping out an e-mail. The font size looks to be seventy-two, about two characters per page. But the point is, he's approaching the century mark and still typing e-mails.

He gives me his usual raised-fist salutation. "Give me one second to finish this up," he says.

My grandfather is a remarkable man. His name is Theodore Kheel, and he has the relentless energy and hearty build of Theodore Roosevelt, for whom he was named. If I want to feel insecure, I need only think about his CV.

His job was a lawyer. But that doesn't begin to describe his range. He worked as a labor mediator, helping to resolve hundreds of strikes—transit workers, bakers, conductors, you name it. He supported the civil rights movement and threw fund-raisers for Martin Luther King Jr. He owned a midget-pony dealership. Well, that last one didn't work out so well.

But the point is, he continues to be involved in an absurd number of projects. He promotes education in rural areas via computerized lectures. He's building an eco-friendly hotel in the Caribbean. He encourages sustainable cuisine and fights overpopulation (though he did have six kids before he converted to that cause).

Naturally, in the last couple of years, he's slowed down. But not totally. At age ninety-two, he started a campaign to make the New York subways and buses free, arguing in Op-eds that it would ease traffic congestion. He wrote op-eds and appeared on the news.

He is not going gentle. And that's no doubt one of the secrets to his longevity. The MacArthur Study of Successful Aging—a respected eight-year-long study of more than one thousand New Englanders—concluded one of the keys is to stay active, connected, involved, and cognitively challenged. You can retire, but you must find something you're passionate about in your retirement. You need some reason to wake up in the morning.

My grandfather shuffles over to join me at the table. He's

stooped over, but he still has a full head of hair. His eyebrows are thick, shaped like arrows that point to the ceiling.

We eat our meal unhurriedly. I've brought my shrimp cocktail fork, which I use to spear a salad. Usually, when he's finished with lunch, my grandfather smacks his hand on the table. But we've been chatting and dining for an hour, and so far there's no hand-smacking. We would make those slow-food Europeans proud.

We talk about mass transit and the legacy of highway booster Robert Moses (my grandfather is not a fan). We discuss the movie he watched last night: one of his all-time favorites, *Inherit the Wind*, based on the life of another accomplished lawyer, Clarence Darrow.

"Did you ever meet Clarence Darrow?" I ask.

My grandfather shakes his head.

"But I did see him speak once at City College," he says.

"You remember anything he said?"

"I do remember."

"And?"

"Well, it was about the sheer improbability that we even exist. The strange fact that out of millions of people in the world, your mother and father met and decided to get married to each other. And out of the millions of sperm, that the one with your genes was the one that made it to the egg and fertilized the egg. I'll never forget it."

It's a little weird to hear your ninety-four-year-old grandfather talk about sperm. But it's still a great point. We should be amazed we exist at all. We ought to be in a constant state of wonder. Maybe we should spend fifteen minutes on a blueberry after all.

Checkup: Month 1

It's been a month since I began Project Health. Here's where I am: I've lost three pounds. The blue digits on my bathroom scale stop flickering at 169. In Julie's estimation, I've gone from looking four months pregnant to three and a half months. This mindful eating is working, at least a little.

Mindfulness has been the big theme of the month. It's invaded every part of my life. Thanks to reading piles of books about health, I've become excruciatingly aware of all my body parts.

When I breathe, I picture the tiny alveoli sacs in my lungs swelling with air. As I type, I visualize the stringlike flexor muscles tugging on my finger bones. As I eat, I imagine the pancreas squirting out its red, enzyme-filled juice, which swarms the peanut butter in the small intestine.

It's a mixed blessing, this mindfulness. Because with it comes anxiety. Lots of it.

I'm more aware of all the horrible ways my body can malfunction. The Centers for Disease Control lists hundreds of diseases, running alphabetically from abdominal aortic aneurysm (a ballooning of the aorta) to zygomycosis (a fungal infection). I watched a TED talk from a doctor who said that our bodies are made of 300 trillion cells, and each of these cells is constantly replicating, and it just takes one of those replications to go slightly awry and a cancer is born. My mother warned me this would happen. She told me the story—which is only half apocryphal—that med students panic their first year when they learn all the diseases. It's not until the second year that they learn the cures.

I'm more aware of my body's many imperfections, the aching lower back, the receding gums, the posture of an exhausted marathoner in the twenty-fifth mile.

I'm more aware of all the many, many changes I have to make to be optimally healthy. That fifty-three-page to-do list I keep on my desk, it haunts me.

My overall strategy is to emphasize one body part at a time. That said, whenever there's an opportunity, I'm also checking off items on the list—no matter which body part is my focus that day.

Last week, for instance, I passed by a plant shop, and stopped in to buy an Areca palm, a task on the fourth page of the list. It's supposedly good for air quality. Unfortunately, its fronds engulfed our entire living room. The boys had to eat dinner hunched over to avoid the branches. Julie made me return it. I replaced it with five smaller plants known, poetically enough, as mother-in-law's tongue (they got their name because of the sharpness of the leaves). Mother-in-law's tongue also effectively cleans the air, according to a NASA study.

But there are hundreds of things left to do to. I have to start sleeping longer. I have to eat better and stop swiping mac 'n cheese and pizza crusts off my kids' plates. And exercise. Aside from an occasional quarter-mile jog in the park, which wipes me out for the next two days, I haven't yet begun to sweat. That's got to end. Or to start.

Chapter 2

The Heart

The Quest to Get My Blood Pumping

I'VE NEVER BEEN A FAN of the gym. I haven't worked out at a gym my entire adult life, a fact Julie finds deeply upsetting. I have several arguments to justify this.

Argument 1: The Jim Fixx argument.

Here we have perhaps the most classic line of reasoning against exercise, and against healthful living in general. I've heard it often, and I've repeated it just as often. It goes like this:

Jim Fixx—the man who helped start the modern fitness revolution, the author of the 1977 classic *The Complete Book of Running*—died at age fifty-two. He collapsed of a heart attack after his daily run in Vermont. So why bother? You never know when death will take you.

The brilliant comic Bill Hicks—who himself died young, at age

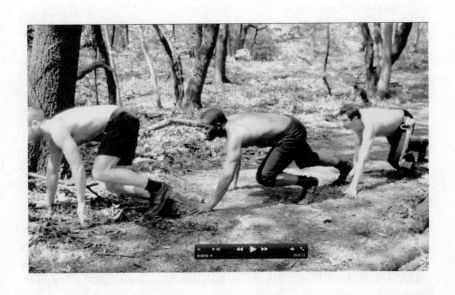

thirty-two, of pancreatic cancer—had a famous bit about Jim Fixx. He imagines an angry Fixx in the afterlife grumbling that he jogged every morning, ate nothing but tofu, and swam five hundred laps a day, and now he's dead. Whereas hard-living actor Yul Brynner drank, chain-smoked, and had young women stroking his "cue-ball head" every night of his life. And he's dead, too. At which point the frustrated Fixx utters a long, stretched-out "shiiiit."

My friend Paul gave me his own version of this argument recently. Actually, he whispered it to me, because he didn't want our wives—both gym fanatics—to overhear us. "Think about it. An hour a day. That's three hundred hours a year. That's three thousand hours in ten years. Think of all the crops that could be planted in that time. Think of all the community service that could be done. And you're extending your life. Why? So you can have five more years of drooling in a bucket?"

Argument 2: In the end, medical advances will save us.

The old long bet. It's another favorite of mine. My friend and former intern Kevin—who is just as bad an influence as Paul—put it this way: "I don't smoke, but I would consider starting. Because it takes, what? Thirty years to get lung cancer. And by the time I get cancer, they'll just give you a gene-coated nano-robot pill and it'll fix it in five minutes."

I think about this point often, because medicine is moving at mach speeds: By the time I'm morbidly obese, they'll probably have a weight-control pill or pineapple-flavored shake to fix it. By the time my teeth have become rotten yellow nubs, you'll be able to grow flawless new bicuspids from stem cells.

In 2010, a Harvard lab headed by Dr. Ronald DePinho actually *reversed* aging in mice. They did it with an enzyme called "telomerase," which acts like little protective caps on the ends of chromosomes. The caps stop the chromosomes from wearing out, a major cause of aging. In ten years, who knows, they might have a human version. Health saints and health sinners might have equal life spans.

Argument 3: Gyms are germ-saturated disease vectors.

As a mild OCD sufferer, I'm a sucker for the microbial argument. Do I want to pick up a dumbbell that has been pawed by a thousand sweaty palms before me? The National Athletic Trainers' Association addresses this topic in a delightfully nauseating paper. It says skin infections from gyms and sports are common, and account for half of the infectious diseases suffered by athletes. They list such unpleasantries as MRSA, athlete's foot, jock itch, boils, impetigo, herpes simplex, and ringworm. As the *New York Times* warned in a headline, BE SURE EXERCISE IS ALL YOU GET AT THE GYM.

So these have been my excuses, the lard-assed devils on my shoulder. And they are somewhat compelling arguments.

But this year, I'm going to have to ignore this thinking. Or shoot the arguments down in my head. Which I can do. After all, Jim Fixx is just one data point, right? Exercise increases life span in general. And being in shape is pleasurable in its own right, so if I eat deep-fried Mars bars and wait around for medical advances, I'm depriving myself of feeling good. Exercise also increases efficiency in everyday life, so I'll be able to plant more crops, think more clearly, and do more community service.

Plus, almost every reputable source recommends regular exercise. Exercise, exercise, exercise. I've read it a thousand times. It cuts down on heart disease and cancer. It's soothes stress and improves concentration. It's like Prozac and Lipitor and Adderall combined. Surprisingly, it doesn't seem to do much for weight loss, partly because a good workout makes us hungry, and we end up bingeing.

But the other benefits? Well documented.

The big debate is over how much and what kind of exercise. And that turns out to be a heated debate indeed.

The Institute of Medicine—an arm of the National Academy of Sciences devoted to evidence-based medicine—recommends "60 minutes of daily moderate intensity physical activity (e.g., walking/jogging at 3 to 4 miles/hour) or shorter periods of more vigorous exertion (e.g., jogging for 30 minutes at 5.5 miles/hour)."

Dr. Oz in his book *You: An Owner's Manual* lets us off easier: To stay young, he suggests twenty minutes of aerobic exercise three times a week, plus a bit of weight lifting. After that, he writes, exercise raises your age, because of the wear and tear on the body. Twenty minutes three times a week. For this, I love Dr. Oz.

There are studies in favor of long-distance running. And there are other studies that say distance running scars the heart.

There's also a growing number of researchers who recommend interval training—lots of walking sprinkled with quick sprints. And still others who dismiss aerobic exercise altogether and say we should focus exclusively on weight training until we reach excruciating muscle failure. But I'll get to that later.

For starters, I'm going to try the Institute of Medicine's daily exercise regimen, blending aerobics and weights. And I'll be confronting my demons and joining the 45 million Americans who belong to a gym.

Losing My Gym Virginity

I choose a gym called Crunch because it is two blocks away from my apartment. Laziness—not a healthy mind-set, I know.

It's a pretty basic, bare-bones gym. The only gimmick is that it's known for its kooky classes, such as pole dancing. (Incidentally, the word "gymnasium" comes from the ancient Greek for "place to be naked," so you could argue pole dancing is actually quite true to gym's roots.)

I'm assigned a trainer named Tony Willging. He's a big man with a shaved head and a tribal tattoo on his arm. He wears a tight black T-shirt that shows off his chest. I tell him I'm writing a book on being superhealthy, and I need to bulk up. I want pecs that would fill a set of B-cups. (Not the manliest way to put it, I suppose.)

"I can do that," says Tony. "But that's not necessarily the same thing as being in shape."

He says healthiness isn't about size. It's overall body condition.

"The thing is," I tell him, "I want before-and-after photos. Like the ones you see in ads for protein shakes."

"Let me tell you something," says Tony. "Those aren't all they're cracked up to be."

At this point, Tony lets me in on a fitness industry secret. Those glossy time-lapse photos are often snapped not months apart, not weeks apart, but . . . on the exact same day. Shave the chest, slather oil on the pecs, suck in the gut, and ta-da, you have a brand-new body. You don't even need Photoshop. Or better yet, the ad company scours the local gyms till they find the most shredded guy around. They snap his photo. They pay him ten thousand dollars to get fat. And then snap his photo a month later. When they print the ad, they simply reverse the "before" and "after" pictures. Point is, it's a lot easier to get out of shape than into it.

This is good information. It takes the pressure off. And if all else fails, I can shave my chest and bathe myself in sesame oil.

On paper, Tony should be the scary, drill-sergeant-like, get-all-up-in-your-grille type of trainer. He looks like he could punch in a windshield with little effort. In his former job, he was a parole officer for murderers and rapists. But Tony's not scary. Quite the opposite. At least to those of us who aren't murderers and rapists, he's gentle and funny, and would rather talk about literary nonfiction than strangleholds.

"Are you up for warming up with a few minutes on the treadmill?" asks Tony, almost apologetically.

Ah, the treadmill. I've always loathed it. Originally, in the 1800s, treadmills were used by horses and prisoners to crush grain (hence the "mill" in treadmill). They also provide us with an almost too-easy Sisyphean metaphor. So there's plenty to hate about the treadmill.

But on I get, and start pattering away—it's only going three miles an hour. And yet, within a hundred steps, I'm panting.

I spend the rest of my training session doing lunges, working with chest press machines, and pumping dumbbells. Thankfully, Tony thinks I'm beyond the lavender-colored dumbbells. But not much beyond. I've got the ten-pounders. I keep looking at the tank-topped man to my left, who is hefting sixty pounders as if they're tubes of toothpaste.

"Don't worry about him," says Tony. "You're doing great."

I leave with a mix of embarrassment and pride. I sweated a bit, not too much. That wasn't so bad, now, was it? And I love the way my arms feel as if they're floating after lifting the weights.

When I get home, Julie hugs me and presents me with a first-day-at-the-gym gift: a PowerBar with a pink candle stuck in it.

"I've waited for this day for years," she says.

For the last decade, Julie has made it her New Year's wish that I join a gym. So for her, my inaugural workout has been one of the highlights of our marriage.

The next day, I had practically no soreness. This bodes well, I thought. What I didn't know is that the soreness often kicks in not the next day, but two days later. (It's called "Delayed Onset Muscle Soreness," and it occurs because of tiny rips in the muscle fibers, especially for those who are out of shape.) And man, did it kick in. I'm walking around like Lurch, straight-legged and angled forward. It takes me a full minute to sit down on the toilet—I have to ease myself onto the seat, clutching onto the sink. Oh, but I'm pleased with the pain. I must be accomplishing something, right?

Going Caveman

I've been hitting the gym a few times a week—and it's been getting slightly less unpleasant—but I want to test other regimens, too. I need to be an exercise omnivore this year. So I've decided to sample the polar opposite of the indoor-gym workout. I'm going to try out the Caveman Workout, which is all about being natural and savage and out in the wilderness. For me, that wilderness is Central Park.

This Sunday, I will join five other men as we toss boulders and run barefoot through Manhattan's own nature preserve.

The caveman movement—or the Paleo movement, as practitioners prefer it to be called—is still somewhat fringe, but it's been gaining traction. The idea is simple. Our bodies evolved for millions of years to eat and exercise a certain way. Then, in relatively recent history, everything changed. Ten thousand years ago, humans started farming. A couple of hundred years ago, we began sitting at our desks all day. For total health, the proponents argue, we need to go back to the old ways—exercising in nature and eating like cavemen.

It's an easy trend to mock. My friends have done so relentlessly: "Is part of the workout dragging women by their hair?" "What was the life expectancy of the caveman? Twenty-eight years? Good luck with that." (Actually, the length of their life span is debatable.)

I'm skeptical of much of the caveman dogma—especially the parts about the meat-heavy diet. I'll get to that later. But I don't think the Paleos should be dismissed. They have some good ideas, too. It's clear that our bodies *were* built for another time. So I want to give this workout a shot.

The man behind the caveman workout is a thirty-nine-year-old Frenchman named Erwan Le Corre, whose company is called MovNat, short for Mouvement Naturel.

He holds workshops around the world—from West Virginia to Thailand—and today he's in New York. We meet at 108th Street and Central Park West at an entrance to the park.

Erwan bounds up wearing black shorts and a sporty zip-up sweater. He's ridiculously good-looking, in a leading-man-in-a-1950s-MGM-movie way: A razor jaw, perfectly coiffed. Sandy brown hair, muscles that are well defined, though not steroidy.

"This is a great place," he says, with a strong French accent, as he scans the scene. "Very natural. Very primal." He runs up the hill to scout out the best patch of trees and rocks.

I wait on the corner with two other cavemen:

One is John Durant, a twenty-six-year-old Harvard grad with dark shoulder-length hair and blue camouflage shorts. The other is Vlad Averbukh, a twenty-nine-year-old with an accent from his native Uzbekistan. Vlad has short red hair, a short red beard, and when not running wild, drives a red Smart Car.

John and Vlad know each other well, having both appeared in a *New York Times* article on the caveman movement.

They chat amiably for a few minutes. Then Vlad starts pressing John on doctrinal differences. Vlad thinks that Paleos should be eating raw meat. His diet includes a lot of raw grass-fed beef and internal organs. John thinks fire was invented much earlier, and cooking your meat is just fine.

"What are your sources?" Vlad asks John.

John sighs. "I don't want to have this debate now."

Vlad seems annoyed, and walks off. I get the feeling Vlad is the fundamentalist caveman, and John is the reform caveman.

Erwan is ready. We leave our shirts in a pile near a rock. It's a brisk day, and the sun apparently wants some privacy, because it refuses to come out from behind some clouds. I clasp myself in a self-hug, hoping to warm up.

"Why do we go bare-chested?" asks Erwan as he stands on a rock. "It's better for us. It toughens us up physically, which toughens us up mentally. It helps us adapt."

There are five of us total, including an African-American caveman named Roshi. Hanging on the sidelines are not one but *two* foreign TV shows taping segments on Erwan: a German show, and a French show, the latter of which, of course, was produced by a black-clad woman whose mouth was never without a lit cigarette.

We jog in place to keep warm.

Vlad leans into me and says, "I'm glad you're here. Because otherwise I would be the least built of everyone."

He glances at my chest again to make sure.

"Uh, thanks?" I say.

"I didn't mean that as an insult. I am just stating facts."

I once wrote an article on a movement called Radical Honesty, where practitioners remove the filter between the brain and the mouth. The article's headline was I THINK YOU'RE FAT. It was an extremely unpleasant experience. I wonder if Vlad is a member of that group, too.

Erwan gives us a preworkout talk on the importance of exercising out in nature. He points to the rocks and hills and uneven ground. "This is better than a gym. It's adaptive for our bodies and our brains."

"You never have this in a gym, because there you do one muscle, then another muscle."

He mimes a biceps curl.

"It's not only inefficient, it's boring."

Our first exercise will be running. We go in single file, crunching through the leaves, dodging broken bottles and jutting rocks.

We run as Erwan instructed. Or at least try. We're supposed to run elegantly, like an animal. Keep the muscles relaxed, lean forward, and let gravity pull you ahead. Don't stomp—take short steps and land lightly on your toes. Don't pump your arms, just let them dangle naturally by your side.

It feels the exact opposite of natural to me, who is used to my old arm-pumping, foot-stomping running. But maybe it'll become natural.

As we round a tree, I step on a glass splinter, barely suppressing a yelp. I don't tell anyone, as I don't want to be the whiner. When we come full circle, we stop to catch our breath.

"How much do you run every day?" Vlad asks Erwan.

"I don't believe in spreadsheets or clocking my heart rate. I do what feels natural and primal. One day I might run five minutes. Another day I might run three hours without stopping."

For our next exercise, we get more primal. We get down on all fours and clamber along a forty-foot fallen log. The idea is to move as if you're a tiger stalking prey.

"It's almost like swimming on the log," says Erwan. "You keep all your muscles relaxed."

Erwan hops on the log, his back flat, and prowls away.

We all get on. It's tricky. My foot keeps slipping, and it's a strain on my shoulders. I try to prowl like a tiger, but end up scurrying like a monkey.

We dismount, and Erwan gives us another pep talk. "In yoga, they say that the mind and body are in touch." He does a mocking California-surfer-dude accent here—or at least a California surfer dude from Provence. "That's fine. But that's not enough. You need to have a mind-body-*nature* connection."

At this point, the TV producers want a shot of John and Erwan interacting with nature by climbing a tree. So Vlad, Roshi, and I have some free time to hang around and chat.

"What's your body fat?" Vlad asks. "My guess is it's eighteen percent."

I tell him I haven't measured it in a bit.

"You have a lot of intravascular fat—fat in between the muscles. If you were a cow, I could make a lot of tallow out of you."

"Uh-huh."

I know I should be angry. So far Vlad has insulted my body twice in the span of a half hour. But there's something disarming—maybe even charming—about his complete lack of social graces. He's like my five-year-old.

The talk turns to diet, as it often does in caveman circles. Vlad extols the virtue of raw grass-fed beef.

"I've found a great supplier of cow brains," he says.

Roshi is interested. "Will you e-mail me the info?"

"Don't you get sick from eating raw food?" asks the German TV producer.

"No, I haven't yet. No worms. Also, in France, parasites are sometimes used in medicine. So it's possible we have a symbiotic relationship with them."

Over the summer, Vlad says, he smushed a bunch of insects together and had them for a meal. "A lot of protein," he said.

As you might imagine, Vlad has no patience for vegans. He's dated a couple over the years. "I converted one to Paleo on the first date—but it didn't work out."

The lack of women in the Paleo movement is a recurring source of frustration. Vlad tells how he had a date over to his apartment, but she left because she thought the bathroom was too dirty. Vlad disagrees with her.

For the first time, I feel a bit bad for Vlad. I want to tell him that it might be easier to date if he was a little more flexible with his no-hygiene-products rule. He won't use deodorant or toothpaste. "I will floss my teeth because chimps have been known to floss their teeth."

For the next exercise, someone suggests lifting a boulder, but we have trouble finding large rocks. Erwan thinks it would be better if all of us carried a log on our shoulders.

The French TV producer is talking quickly and with seeming concern to Erwan. I can't understand what she's saying, but I do hear the word *dangereux.*

Erwan shakes his head. "*C'est pas dangereux.*"

Hmm. That doesn't sound good. We get in line, and on the count of three, we heave a log onto our shoulders, It's as thick as a telephone pole, and my knees buckle a bit before I regain my balance.

After we stagger forward about ten yards, Erwan shouts that it's time to toss it back onto the ground. We all grunt, and the log thumps to the dirt.

Vlad approaches Erwan.

"What can I do about this?" Vlad asks. He points to his shoulder, which he's scratched up while carrying the log.

Erwan shrugs. Maybe aloe vera, someone suggests.

"Use the blood of your enemies," says John.

We all laugh, except for Vlad. I feel the tribe fracturing. I'm worried for Vlad. I want him to censor himself and get back on the good side of the alpha males, but I don't know if he can.

Erwan lifts his foot and points to a bloody toe that he got while climbing the tree.

"Cuts and scratches help renew the body," he says.

Our final exercise will be sprinting. In Paleolithic times, the theory goes, there wasn't a lot of leisurely jogging. There was walking, then sprinting. You'd sprint from a hungry tiger, or sprint to catch an antelope.

We start on a bike path, we pack of shirtless guys. Erwan gives a signal, and we all sprint across the street at a diagonal angle, dodging bikers and in-line skaters, pumping our legs, then hopping over a short wooden fence on the other side.

Erwan smiles widely. "You feel alive? That's the way to work out. No warm-up. Just sprinting!"

You know what? I do feel alive. That was fantastic. Liberating. I can feel my heart expanding and contracting. I can feel my skin tingle.

A gray-haired women approaches us to ask us why five half-naked men are sprinting through the park. We try to explain. "Oh, I thought you were robbing someone," she says matter-of-factly, and then leaves.

We walk back across the street to prepare for another speed run.

"Can we start on smoother pavement?" asks Vlad. "This hurts my feet."

"Listen," says Erwan coolly. "Toughen up."

Everyone laughs, except Vlad.

"For someone who boils their meat, that's talking pretty tough," Vlad shoots back.

Vlad turns to John: "And I can tell you trim your chest hair."

"I'm not sure what your fascination is with my chest hair," responds John to a tense silence.

We sprint through the bikers again, jumping over the fence. Erwan and John are ahead. I edge out Vlad by a couple of feet—a fact he ignores. "I'm glad you're here because you're as slow as I am, and I didn't want to be the slowest one."

He does make it hard to feel bad for him.

And that's it. Three hours of huffing and puffing in New York's woods. I'm cold and tired, and I have to take care of my cavekids.

As we say good-bye, Erwan asks again about the premise my book.

"It's about me trying to be the healthiest man alive."

"I'm not trying to give you a hard time," Erwan says, with a smile. "But I am *being* the healthiest man alive. Not trying. *Being.*"

When I get home, I spend twenty minutes digging the glass splinter out of my toe while telling Julie about Vlad and his barrage of insults.

"So will you be running around with a loincloth from now on?"

No. Probably not. But the caveman workout shouldn't be dismissed. For one thing, I have to concede that Erwan has a point about exercising under the sky.

I've always preferred the indoor life—to quote Woody Allen, I'm at two with nature—but that's not going to work this year. Recent research shows that just being outside improves your health, at least for those without debilitating hay fever. A Nippon Medical School study showed that two-hour walks in a forest caused a 50 percent spike in natural killer cells, a powerful immune cell.

A 2010 study asked 280 subjects in Japan to take strolls in both the park and the city. After the nature walks, the participants showed lower "concentrations of the stress hormone cortisol, lower pulse rate, lower blood pressure." Strolling through parks is apparently a popular hobby in Japan, and goes by the poetic and slightly racy name of "forest bathing."

What's so great about the great outdoors? One theory is that plants release a chemical called "phytoncides." Plants use the chemical to protect themselves from decay, but it may benefit people, too.

It may be simpler than that. It may be that the very sight of nature calms us down. There's a famous 1984 University of Delaware study in which patients recovering from gallbladder surgery stayed in different hospital rooms. Some had a view of a green field, some had a view of a brick wall. The ones with the natural view recovered more quickly and required less powerful painkillers. They even liked their nurses more.

Exercise and Old Age

A few days later, I ran through Central Park to visit my grandfather. I had to stop a couple of times to catch my breath, but I made the mile and half jog without collapsing, which is an improvement.

When I got to his apartment, my grandfather asked me about my health quest. I told him about the cavemen, which made him chuckle.

He was sitting in his recliner, where he spends most of his day, his feet propped up and swollen from poor circulation. Walking is hard because of a slipped disk. It's strange to see him this way. Unlike me, my grandfather was athletic for almost all of his life—tennis, running, biking, Frisbee. He was the only person I knew who had a rowing machine in his home. And pogo sticks.

Even in his eighties, he swam in the rough Atlantic surf. He'd wade in and a wave would smack him. He'd stumble momentarily, but then plow ahead, get smacked again, plow ahead.

When I was a kid, he'd play Ping-Pong, and to make the game fair, he'd get down on his knees. He'd take me on bike rides, powering up the hills on the same orange Kabuki ten-speeder that he owned for decades. He'd often ride sitting straight up, clasping his hands behind his head. Not the best safety role model, but I loved it.

My late grandmother was obsessed with exercise as well, constantly nudging me to stop lolly gagging, as she put it.

"I thought of Grandma the other day," I tell my grandfather. "She always told me that orchestra conductors lived a long time because they moved their arms so much. This book I'm reading says there may be truth to that."

My grandfather smiles, and waves an imaginary baton.

"A wise woman," he says.

My grandmother died six years ago, just short of their sixty-eighth anniversary. Theirs was a good marriage. Not a perfect one. But good.

He loved to tease her. At the dinner table, if the conversation turned to somebody's upcoming nuptials, he'd go into the office and retrieve his *Bartlett's Quotations*. He'd open it to George Bernard Shaw's passage on marriage and read it to the table:

When two people are under the influence of the most violent, most insane, most delusive and most transient of passions, they are required to swear that they will remain in that excited, abnormal and exhausting condition until death do them part.

Then he'd giggle until he shook.

"Oh, Ted," Grandma would respond, laughing. She got back at

45

him, though. Eventually, she tore out the page and those readings came to an abrupt end.

Another time, we were out to dinner at an Italian place near their apartment. During a pause, my grandfather turned to me and asked, "How do you think the *New York Post* is going to play it?"

"Play what?" I asked.

"How will they play it when they find out Grandma's pregnant?"

Then he'd giggle until he shook.

"Oh, Ted," Grandma responded.

But even when teasing, he was devoted. He still had at least some of that insane and delusive passion that he had when they met while students at Cornell in 1932 (he climbed up the side of her building to see her because men weren't allowed inside the women's dorm). Even to the end, he still held her hand when they walked. Or occasionally, he'd goose her ("Oh, Ted").

"She was the greatest woman I ever knew," he told me over lunch, a few weeks after she died. His eyes shined with tears.

Their marriage was likely as important to his longevity as his constant aerobic activity. Studies have shown that a good marriage is a boon to your health. It's been associated with a lower rate of heart attacks—as well as of pneumonia, cancer, and dementia.

I find the marriage/health link massively unfair. Nature is being a bit of a sadistic bastard. So you found your soul mate? Let's reward you with a long life and freedom from sickness. Haven't been lucky enough to find that special someone? Sorry. You'll probably die sooner. It reminds me of how highly paid celebrities get free cars, shoes, and jewelry. Those of us without $15-million-per-movie contracts have to actually buy things.

Yet whether I like it or not, the statistics point to marriage as healthy. Though I should qualify that. As Tara Parker-Pope writes in her book *For Better: The Science of a Good Marriage*, staying in a bad marriage is terrible for your health. "One recent study suggests that a stressful marriage can be as bad for the heart as a regular smoking habit," she writes.

But why do good marriages help? Pope lists a few of the more common theories:

- Married folks are less likely to engage in unhealthy behaviors such as excessive drinking and staying out late.
- Marriage comes with familial and social ties that lower stress.
- And married men are more likely to visit the doctor, thanks to their wives' pestering.

That last one isn't a trivial point. I wonder if my grandfather—a typically stoic man—would have gone to the doctor without my grandmother's urging. Even now she's looking out for him, in a way. As she was dying in the hospital, she pleaded with her kids to take care of their father—and each other.

After an hour of chatting with my grandfather, I said good-bye. I was planning on running back across Central Park, but an empty cab pulled up right in front of me at a red light. And what can I say? I'm a weak man.

Outwitting Myself

I wish I enjoyed exercising more. Julie—owner of an impressive collection of bike shorts and sports bras—loves the gym. She looks forward to it in much the same way I look forward to reading on the couch while she's at the gym.

In the bestseller *Born to Run*, Christopher McDougall writes about tapping into humans' innate and infectious "joy of running."

With rare exceptions (like after that sprint through the park during the caveman workout), I don't feel the joy of running. I feel the joy of lounging. Maybe I'll grow to love physical exertion over time, like spouses in arranged marriages learn to adore each other. But for now, running and I are barely on speaking terms.

So I have to get clever. My only chance is to outwit myself into exercising. One tactic is to leave my shorts and sneakers by the door at night. Research shows you're more likely to work out if you give yourself visual cues, such as this one. (I've found it helpful, except when Julie puts away my shorts, thinking I'm just being sloppy.)

My favorite tactic, though, is an admittedly unorthodox method I came up with after reading about "egonomics."

Egonomics is a theory by a Nobel Prize–winning economist named Thomas Schelling. Schelling proposes that we essentially have two selves. Those two selves are often at odds. There's the present self, that wants that frosted apple strudel Pop-Tart. And the future self, that regrets eating that frosted apple strudel Pop-Tart.

The key to making healthy decisions is to respect your future self. Honor him or her. Treat him or her like you would treat a friend or a loved one.

But the future self—that's so abstract, I thought. What if I made my future self more concrete? So I downloaded an iPhone app called HourFace that digitally ages your photo. I did it with a picture of myself, and, well, the results were alarming. My face sagged and became splotchy—I looked like I had some sort of biblical skin disease.

I've printed the photo out and taped it to my wall, alongside my Carl Sagan quotation about skeptical open-mindedness. And you know? It works. When I'm wavering about whether to lace up my running sneakers or not, I'll catch sight of Old A.J. Respect your elder, as disturbing looking as he may be. This workout is for him.

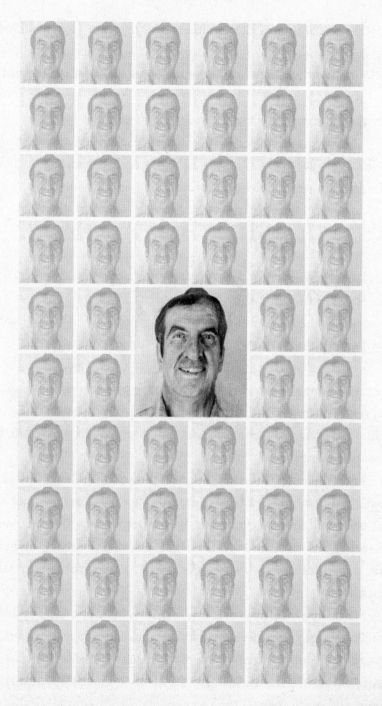

The future self needs to be around for my sons. They deserve to know him.

I thought Julie would dismiss my egonomics, but she found it intriguing.

"Can you age me?" she asked. When I showed her photo to her, she burst out laughing and said she looked like Dustin Hoffman. That's inspiring, she said. On the rare times she doesn't feel like exercising, she'll do it for Dustin.

Checkup: Month 2

Weight: 167
Hours of sleep per night: 6 (not good)
Visits to the gym: 12 (should have been more)
Bench press: 55 pounds, 15 reps

I only lost a pound this month, but that's because I'm gaining muscle weight. Or at least that's what I tell myself as I flex in my bathroom mirror searching for any microscopic changes to my biceps and chest.

I'm still doing my best to control portions. Still using my kids' cartoon dinosaur plates at home. At restaurants, I transfer half my entrée onto the smaller butter plate, and get the other half in a doggie bag. My chew-per-mouthful ratio is ten to one, which is decent, if not great. I carry my little blue-and-white shrimp fork in my back pocket wherever I go—which has resulted in tiny holes in the back of my jeans, as well as several puzzled waiters who returned the fork to me after I accidentally left it on the plate.

So the portion size is respectable. But what should I *put in* those portions? I'm still struggling with what constitutes a healthy menu.

This month, at the very least, I pledged to cut down on sugar, since almost everyone agrees it's poisonous in large doses. But the stuff is so sneaky. Case in point: I was at Newark Airport—on my way to Los Angeles for an *Esquire* article—and I spotted a little kiosk called Healthy Garden. That sounds promising, I think to myself. So I wander over only to find: highly salted Chex mix, plastic containers of gummi bears and Swedish fish, "Grandma's" chocolate chip cookie (I'm assuming from the ingredients that Grandma has a Ph.D. in chemistry from CalTech), and a "healthy mix" of fruit and nuts. The "healthy mix" contained some decent stuff, like walnuts and almonds. But it also had banana chips, which included refined cane sugar, coconut oil, and best of all, banana flavor. When you need to add banana flavor to bananas, there's something askew with the world of food.

My sugar woes aside, I do feel slightly healthier overall. Less logy, more energetic. As if my body used to be cloudy and smog-filled (think Beijing), and now it's only moderately polluted (maybe Houston). I like climbing a flight of stairs without my heart thumping like a cartoon animal in love.

But is that sensation worth all the hours at the gym and the dietary restrictions and extra showers? I'm not convinced. Maybe I need a break. For my next body part, I'll do something that doesn't require additional sweating or hunger pangs.

photo tk

Chapter 3

The Ears

The Quest for Quiet

WE TOOK OUR THREE SONS to Benihana for dinner tonight. It's
their favorite restaurant, thanks to the unbeatable combination of
airborne food and machete-size knives.

But healthy it's not.

First, there's the food, an orgy of salt and grease. Second, there's
the smoke from all the grills, which fills the room and is eye-
rubbingly thick, what I imagine it'd be like in a Charles de Gaulle
Airport lounge circa 1965.

But what I notice tonight is the noise. The hiss of the soy sauce
on the grill, the escalating chatter of the crowd. And my sons. God
love them, but my sons are loud beyond comprehension. (Whenever I ask my son Zane to be quiet because his mom is napping,
he'll walk by her room shouting, "TIPTOE! TIPTOE!")

Tonight, they're each carrying around a little plastic trumpet they were given at a friend's birthday. Interesting choice for a party favor. How about handing my kids a pack of Marlboros and some razors? I might have preferred that.

They've been tooting their horns since we left the gymnastics-themed party, so I feel like I've been followed around by my own private South African soccer game. Right before the appetizers come, we finally pry the ghastly things from their hands.

My goodness, it's a loud world. I've started to become aware of this more and more during my health project. Just spend an hour listening. The chirping text messages, the droning airplanes, the flatulent trucks, the howling cable pundits, the chiming MacBooks, the crunching orange foodlike snacks.

Thanks to my reading, I know that noise is not a minor nuisance. No, noise is one of the great underappreciated health hazards of our time, damaging not just our hearing, but our brain and heart. It's the secondhand smoke of our ears. Some say even worse, like aural mustard gas.

Noise pollution doesn't get the attention of A-list diseases. There are no parades or ribbons or celebrity spokespeople. But there are a handful of brave, slightly eccentric crusaders raising their voices against the onslaught of noise. One of them—the Mother Jones of the movement—is a psychology professor at the City University of New York named Arline Bronzaft. She agrees to let me visit at her upper East Side apartment.

A petite woman with short brown hair, Bronzaft lives in an apartment that is, appropriately, shielded from most traffic noise. It's filled with photos of her beloved Yankees and her equally beloved grandson, who recently had a nice, restrained five-piece band at his bar mitzvah. "My daughter said to the musicians, 'If you make it too loud, my mother will disinherit me,'" says Bronzaft.

We sit in her kitchen to talk noise.

What's the problem with this high-decibel world?

"The most obvious one is hearing loss," she says.

Around 26 million adults are walking around with noise-induced hearing loss. And with our omnipresent earbuds, that number is bound to rise.

Even without earbuds, we naturally lose hearing as we age, as the sensory hair cells inside the cochlea erode. Babies can hear forty thousand cycles per second, while the average adult can hear at twenty thousand cycles per second. Our ability to hear higher registers goes first, which means that the voices of women and children are silenced sooner, as if God were W. C. Fields.

Hearing loss is bad enough, but it's not even the most pressing problem. Noise has a surprisingly potent effect on our stress level, cardiovascular system, and concentration. Just go back to our Paleo ancestor for a minute. In caveman times, a loud noise signaled a threat—an angry mastodon, perhaps. So noise activates the infamous fight-or-flight response: high adrenaline and high blood pressure. Nowadays, we're bombarded by loud noises almost all day long, meaning our fight-or-flight instinct gets little downtime. One review found that people who work noisy jobs suffered two to three times the heart problems as those who work in quiet settings. In his book *In Pursuit of Silence*, George Prochnik cites a former World Health Organization official who estimates—with perhaps a bit of alarmism—that "45,000 fatal heart attacks per year may be attributable to noise-related cardiovascular strain."

Something starts whirring in Bronzaft's kitchen.

"What's that sound?" I ask.

"The refrigerator," she says. "When I found out it made that noise, I was shocked."

Noise harms the ears and the heart—but it also wreaks havoc on the brain.

Our wise founding fathers knew this back in the 1700s. "When they wrote the Constitution in Independence Hall in Philadelphia, they realized noise was going to disrupt them because the horses and wagons would clatter over the cobblestones," Bronzaft says. "So they packed dirt on the cobblestones to lessen the noise of passing traffic."

That's right. Noise is unpatriotic. (And quite possibly fascist. I read a quote from Hitler that he "couldn't have won Germany without a bullhorn.")

Bronzaft was one of the first to show scientifically that noise messes with the mind. In 1970, she was working as a transportation adviser to the mayor of New York, helping to design the subway map. She wasn't even focused on noise pollution. (And oddly, she says that she isn't overly sensitive to noise; she became interested in it as a public health problem.)

She conducted a landmark study at a public school in Manhattan's Washington Heights neighborhood. Some of the classrooms faced directly out on an elevated subway track. Every five minutes the students heard a train rattle by. Other classrooms were tucked on the opposite side of the building, away from the noise. The difference? By the sixth grade, the kids in the quiet classrooms were about one year ahead in reading.

Her conclusions have since been backed up by a pile of other studies, both on students and adults. As George Prochnik writes, even "moderate noise from white-noise machines, air conditioners and background television, for example, can still undermine children's language acquisition."

When Bronzaft started, the antinoise movement was seen somewhere between organic foods and mandatory clothes for Greek sculpture on the kookiness scale. Nowadays, it's edging ever closer to the mainstream. There are more noise-reducing ceilings, altered flight patterns, and warning labels on products. There are activists all over the country tilting at wind turbines, motocross raceways, and leaf blowers. "This is not just a big-city problem," says Bronzaft.

It's been almost two hours. Bronzaft may be antinoise, but she's not the quiet type. She's a talker.

She tells me the plot of her unpublished novel about an old lady killed by her loud neighbors. It's called *For Dying Out Loud*.

"Did my novel have sex in it? Yes, it did. A lot. My daughters couldn't read it. Did it depict noise? Yes. It had murder, it had mystery, but it didn't have a novelist's touch. I'm too academic."

I interrupt Bronzaft to tell her that I have to pick up my kids from school. I say good-bye, catch the bus, and ride home trying to ignore the rumbles and squeaks of traffic.

Listening Carefully

That evening, I pledge to turn down the volume on my life. I start in my kids' room. I dig out all their beeping, screeching, yammering electronic toys, and spend half an hour putting masking tape over the plastic speakers

"What are you doing, Daddy?" asks Lucas.

"Just fixing the broken toys," I half lie.

It was a smashing success, at least from my point of view. You can still hear "Chicken Dance Elmo" demand that we "flap our wings," but he sounds like he's submerged in a bathtub, which is what I'd really like to do to him.

Next up, ear protection. I ordered reusable orange silicone SilentEar earplugs at the Ear Plug Superstore. They worked for a week or so. But I didn't love the feeling of something penetrating my ear hole, so I shelled out for a pair of Bose noise-canceling headphones. They cost a stress-inducing three hundred dollars.

I try them out on a plane to Atlanta, where I'm going on a business trip. I slip them over my ears, click the power switch, and . . . well, the world didn't go silent. I can still hear the dinging seat-belt sign. But the headphones do turn the volume down from a ten to a seven. Life takes on a sort of a dreamy, uterine feel.

In the next few weeks, I start to wear my headphones more and more. They're on my head right now, these big silver-and-black earmuffs. I look like a baggage handler on the tarmac at JFK.

I wear them while working, while picking up my sons from school, while brushing my teeth. People ask, "What are you listening to?" Just the lovely sounds of silence, I say.

Julie has taken to calling me Lionel Richie, because I look like I just walked out of the recording studio for "We Are the World." At least I'm 95 percent sure that's what she calls me. I tend to miss a word here or there, like a bad Skype connection to Ecuador. I'm usually able to cover it up with nods and smiles. Never underestimate the power of the nod and smile.

The headphones aren't fool proof. I recently wore them to a playdate at my friend John's apartment.

"Please take them off," Julie said as we waited for the elevator.

"Why?"

"They're dorky."

"They're the same as sunglasses. They're protecting my ears. Sunglasses protect my eyes. Same idea. Blocking out harmful stimuli. Why are sunglasses cool and earphones dorky?"

"Please take them off."

I acceded.

But this just spurs me to prove to Julie just how perilously loud our lives are, so I order a decibel meter on the Internet. It looks like a rectal thermometer. I carry mine around everywhere, surreptitiously taking it out and testing the air whenever possible.

Here's a sample of my findings. And remember, decibel levels above eighty-five—about the sound of a leaf blower—can cause permanent hearing loss.

Dave & Buster's restaurant/video arcade in Times Square: 102 decibels

New York's C-line subway entering the station: 110

Zane's tantrum about missing the last five minutes of *Bubble Guppies*: 91

Julie in an argument about whether or not I misplaced her *Time* magazine: Unknown.

Whenever I put the decibel meter near her mouth, she refuses to talk. As Werner Heisenberg knew, taking measurements can mess with reality.

Checkup: Month 3

Weight: 168

Push-ups till exhaustion: 34

Walks in the park: 8

Blood pressure: 115/75

According to a University of Manchester study, my headphones might make my food taste better. The study found that background noise dampens our taste buds, which is part of the reason most airline lasagna tastes like Astro Turf.

This finding is good, as I need more incentive to eat healthy food. I'm trying to eat right, but only succeeding in fits and starts.

I downloaded a list of superfoods from Dr. Oz's website, and I go on nutritional binges. I'm on a mission to break my own record for the most superfoods eaten one sitting. My record so far is eight. Yesterday, I spent half an hour making a lunch salad of mango (vitamin C helps prevent periodontal disease), fennel (anti-inflammatory), blueberries (antioxidants, of course), avocados (mono-unsaturated fat), pomegranate seeds (ellagic acid that preserves collagen in skin), dark chocolate shavings, ground kelp, and lentils (good source of zinc). I like this idea of competition as an incentive to healthy eating, even if it's just a competition to break my own record. Maybe games are the way to change our habits. Perhaps the competitive eating circuit could substitute kale for Coney Island hot dogs.

Meanwhile, I'm trying to exercise every day, though I only manage about four times a week. To boast that number, I decided to buy a treadmill off Craigsist for three hundred dollars.

"Where are we going to fit it?" asked Julie.

"The bedroom?" I said.

She paused. "Normally I'm against big machinery in the apartment. But if it'll help you get in shape . . ."

And it *was* helping for a while. I was running two or three miles at 5 mph almost every day. Then we got a call from our downstairs neighbor, Lloyd. Apparently, everyone on the entire fourth floor is in a tizzy. The pounding from my treadmill reverberates from one end of the building to the other. One neighbor wants to know why, every night, the paintings on his walls bounce.

If I were in Bronzaft's novel, I'd be murdered in my sleep. I've had to abandon my treadmill. It sits in my bedroom, a silent reminder of a wasted three hundred dollars.

Back to the gym it is. I can't say that I relish it, but I don't dread it as much as I once did.

There are parts of the gym ritual I find comforting. I like nodding at my fellow regulars, such as the guy who reads the Talmud while on the stationary bike. Or the guy who does biceps curls and then thumps his chest like Tarzan. Or the guy whose workout getup—tube socks and a white headband—makes him look like he stepped out of the 1985 Jamie Lee Curtis movie *Perfect*.

And thank God for Tony. He's supportive, always saying how much improvement I'm making, even if I've been stuck on the fifteen-pound biceps curls for three weeks. He's an understanding mentor, and happy to give me tips on gym etiquette. "You can't let the weights clank down," he says. "It draws negative attention. People think you're weak. On the other hand, if you do a lot of grunting and then clank, that's okay. But you got to plan for it."

So overall, I feel decent. Even good. Perhaps the best I've felt since high school.

But every time I start to edge toward smugness, I read something that stresses me out. The latest study that's obsessing me: It might not matter if I'm exercising for an hour a day. If I'm sitting down for the other sixteen waking hours, I'm almost as unhealthy as ever.

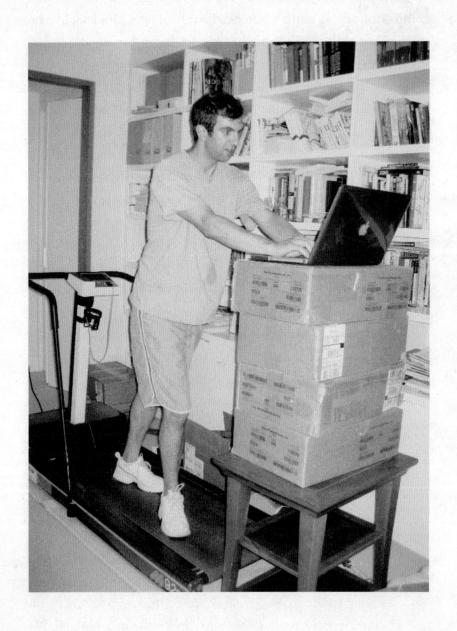

Chapter 4

The Butt

The Quest to Avoid Sedentary Life

FOUR MONTHS IN, I'VE DECIDED it's time to declare war on my Sedentary Life. It's not a war I want to fight. I've never had anything against the Sedentary Life. It suits me just fine. Before Project Health, I sat happily for ten to twelve hours a day. My Aeron chair and my butt were soul mates. I remember complaining to Julie once about the idea of the standing ovation. Is it really necessary? Can't we express our approval for *Wicked* while comfortably seated? Maybe we could raise our arms or bow our heads or stomp our feet.

But the more I read, the more I realize an unfortunate truth: Sitting and staring at screens all day is bad for you. Really bad, like smoking-unfiltered-menthols-while-eating-cheese-coated-lard-and-screaming-at-your-spouse bad. Michelle Obama is right. We need to move. Chairs are the enemy. Sitting puts you at risk for heart disease, diabetes, obesity, and some types of cancer, including colorectal and ovarian.

We weren't built to sit. Never before in history have we been so immobile. According to Harvard professor John Ratey, our Paleolithic forefathers walked eight to ten miles a day. Our grandparents expended an average of three thousand calories a day as opposed to our measly two thousand. According to the book *The Blue Zones*, the cultures with the longest life spans—such as those in Okinawa and Sardinia—move all the time, lugging food up steep hills. (I wish New York had more hills. It's dangerously flat.)

The problem for Americans is that we've Balkanized our lives. We go to the gym for an hour (if we're dutiful) and then sit for the rest of the day. Movement is sealed into an airtight container. When I was twelve, I had a strange fantasy about isolating all of life's activities and batching them together. I wished I could brush my teeth for a month, then be finished with that for the rest of my life. I'd go to the bathroom for two years. Perhaps have sex for six weeks. We live in a less extreme version of my scenario. We sit and sit and sit, then have a burst of movement.

Studies show that even regular gym going can't fully undo the harm of sitting. So my plan is to tear down the wall between exercise and life. I've started doing what I call guerrilla exercise—or what my friend calls contextual exercise. I squeeze physical activity into every nook in my day.

I climb the four flights of stairs to our apartment. "Meet you up there," Julie will say as she hops in the elevator. Once in a while, I'll beat her to our front door and wait there, tapping my watch, looking impatient and trying not to hyperventilate. "Good one," she says as she walks by.

I avoid the People Movers at airports. Yes, I move my own

person. I actually roll my suitcase over the stationary ground. I know! Heroic.

I read one health article that recommended doing pull-ups from the "Don't Walk" sign when waiting at the corner. I tried that. Even my five-year-old was embarrassed for me. So I stopped.

And, in my biggest change yet, I've started to run errands. Literally run them. In normal usage, "running errands" is one of the most euphemistic phrases in the English language. We don't run errands. We walk errands. Or, more often, we drive errands.

But for the past couple of weeks, I've been on a mission of literalness. I run to the drugstore, buy a toothbrush, then run home. I run to the grocery, to the barber, to pick up my kids at school.

Granted, running errands has its downsides. I sweated through my shirt on my way to an *Esquire* meeting. (I now carry an extra stick of deodorant in my bag). It can take longer than doing an errand in a car or bus—though not always, especially if it's a ten-block-or-under errand.

Also, it freaks people out. Grown man in regular clothes aren't supposed to run in public. The other day, I was running down the street—dressed in jeans and a big puffy coat—and a woman pushing a stroller stopped and shouted after me, "Is everything okay?" She probably thought a dirty bomb had just detonated.

Running errands takes an act of will. I have to force my recalcitrant legs to start pumping with a ten-nine-eight countdown. But oh, the upsides. For one thing, it eases the guilt if I skip the gym one day. The world is my gym, I tell myself. And the bags of cereal and orange juice and toothpaste are my dumbbells. And there's a glorious feeling of efficiency—you're multitasking, but in a low-tech and beneficial way that won't frazzle your brain or cause four-car pileups. Running errands also burns more calories than walking the same distance. (Running a mile erases 124 calories for men, while walking a mile only takes 88. So say the studies.)

So that's my new thing, telling Julie "I'm off to run some errands."

Even if I'm not running, I try to avoid sitting. All this antisedentary research has had a weird and unpleasant effect on my psyche. I can no longer rest in peace. The longer I'm seated, the guiltier I feel. After half an hour, I have that same queasy sensation I get from binging on half of a box of Chips Ahoy!

The problem with sitting, as biologist and author Olivia Judson explains, is twofold. The first part is obvious: We burn fewer calories when we're sitting. The second part is more subtle, but perhaps more profound: marathon sitting sessions change our body's metabolism. A molecule called lipase is crucial to helping muscles absorb fat. When we sit, we don't produce lipase, allowing the fat to go off and do naughty things like deposit itself as body fat or clog the arteries.

There are plenty of studies on lipase. To take just one: The University of South Carolina and Pennington Biomedical Research Center compared heart problems in men who spent more than twenty-three hours a week sitting, and those who sat for less than eleven hours. The big sitters had a 64 percent higher chance of fatal heart disease. And the bad news doesn't end there. The sitters weren't slackers. A lot of them went to the gym when they weren't sitting. But their workouts couldn't fully overcome the damage from their desk chair.

So when I'm not moving, I try to stand, which is at least something. As Judson writes, "Compared to sitting, standing in one place is hard work. To stand, you have to tense your leg muscles, and engage the muscles of your back and shoulders; while standing, you often shift from leg to leg. All of this burns energy."

Julie and I went to see *Star Trek* last night, and after forty minutes, I excused myself to stand in the back of the theater.

I felt righteous. Sitting during entertainment? That's for the effete and the weak. I convinced myself I was a descendant of the hardy groundlings, the folks who paid a penny to stand in the dirt pit at Shakespeare's Globe Theatre.

"There are plenty of seats," the usher whispered to me.

"Thanks, I'm good."

I listened to the soothing whir of the projector as he kept a wary eye on me.

Speed Writing

And then . . . there's the desk. The desk is where most of the Crimes of Excessive Sedentary Behavior occur.

Something needed to be done. For a week, I switched to working while standing. I raised my laptop by loading up three cardboard boxes onto my desk. Then I'd stand and peck out e-mails. I heard once that Nabokov wrote his novels standing up, so I was hoping my e-mails would have a *Pale Fire* quality to them.

It didn't go badly. I shifted and rocked a lot. I kind of looked like an Orthodox Jew praying at the Western Wall, but with a MacBook instead of a Torah. I kept a stack of two encyclopedias at my feet so that I could rest one foot on it at a time, a key to comfortable long-term standing.

But the real breakthrough came when I combined the desk and movement.

I kept flashing back to the Execusiser in Woody Allen's *Bananas*. It was a brilliant invention: a desk combined with a workout station. The phone receiver was hooked up to elastic bands, so answering a call resulted in a biceps curl. That kind of thing.

I couldn't find any real-life Execusisers online. I found the next best thing, though: an idea from Dr. James Levine, a researcher at the Mayo Clinic. He thinks we should all have our desks in front of treadmills. We should all walk as we work. Levine has gained a small but loyal following of treadmill desk jockeys. They trade tips and stories on the websites, and coin terms like *"deskercise"* and "iPlod."

You can buy professionally made treadmill desks for four hundred dollars. Or you can jury-rig your own. I chose the latter.

I did so because I already have a treadmill—the one lying fallow thanks to the complaints of my neighbors below. If I *walk* on my treadmill, my neighbors can't protest. It's so civilized, so quiet. I stroll at barely one mile per hour.

I balanced my laptop on top of a wooden box, and I slung a long pole across my treadmill to rest my elbows. This arrangement, by the way, came after about a half-dozen collapsed versions involving dictionaries, filing cabinets, and masking tape. But it works.

I'm on it right now. This chapter has taken about 1.5 miles to write. I want this book to be the first book written mostly on a treadmill.

There are some skeptics. My aunt Marti chided me. She said it's multitasking. She told me I'm not in the moment. Very un-Buddhist. Julie asked me, "Isn't it distracting to type and walk?"

But overall, I'm liking it. In the beginning, it was a little odd. You have to get over the initial hump, that siren call of the chair. But now I found walking while working actually helps hone my focus. When I'm sitting, I'm fidgety. I'm always tempted to stand up and get a snack, use the bathroom, water the plants—anything to avoid working. With my treadmill desk, I'm getting rid of all my nervous energy. Plus, when you're walking, you can't fall asleep. No small thing.

I wonder if the Tread-desk has changed my writing style? Are my sentences more energetic? I can't tell. I do know that I feel more confident and positive when I'm striding along, more likely to answer e-mails with an emphatic "Yes! I would love to go mountain biking in Connecticut, despite the forecast of thunderstorms." So I have to be careful.

Standing in the Presence of the Elderly

I spent some time standing at my grandfather's apartment today. It felt almost natural not to sit. The Old Testament commands us to stand in the presence of the elderly, so it was a nice callback to my days of living biblically. I stand behind my grandfather's cushy brown recliner.

I'm visiting on movie day. My grandfather's former colleague is over, and wants to see a documentary in which my grandfather appeared. My aunt Jane—a lawyer visiting from Maryland—slides in the DVD and presses play. The documentary is about the artist Christo and his Central Park *Gates.* These, as you might remember, consisted of a forest of metal poles draped in orange fabric that appeared in the park in 2005. My grandfather was Christo's lawyer.

I've seen the movie before. But it's a joy to watch it with him. He gets such a kick out of his younger, brasher self.

The movie opens with my grandfather and Christo's first meeting more than thirty years ago. You hear the comically loud clacking of typewriters, and watch as Christo and his wife, Jeanne-Claude, enter my grandfather's office. He's on the phone sounding important ("Good," "Okay" "Let's make sure the record is correct") and nods at them as they settle into chairs.

Eventually he hangs up, puts his index finger on his temple, and listens as this stringy-haired eccentric Bulgarian and his French wife tell him their zany plans. They want to install eighteen thousand gates in Central Park.

My 1979 grandfather practically does a spit take. My 2010 grandfather, watching in his recliner, laughs. "I had never met them before," he says. "I'd barely heard of them. I thought they were nuts."

At meeting's end, he agrees to be their lawyer. He tells them the next step is to petition the Parks Department. My grandfather says, "You've got to think like [the Parks Department]. They're thinking what can go wrong. What'll the Jews say, what'll the Irish say, what'll the Poles say?"

My grandfather worked with the Christos for twenty-six years, seeing them through hundreds of meetings, committees, briefs, and fund-raising events. "I know it'll happen one day," he always said. And then, finally, there it was, this bizarre but beautiful ocean of apricot-colored fabric in Central Park.

The documentary ends with the 2005 unveiling of *The Gates*. You can see my grandfather sitting between the Christos in the backseat of a car, touring Central Park. He's more stooped than his 1979 self, less stooped than his 2010 version, but he still has the ever-present childlike wonder: "Wow. Wow. Wow," he says as they pass by *The Gates*.

My 2010 grandfather smiles and says, "It only took twenty-six years." It really is a remarkable statistic. It's a real lesson in fortitude, optimism, and persistence. The Little Conceptual Art Project That Could.

I've often wondered if my grandfather's unflagging determination and optimism is a key to his longevity. Some studies point to yes: A fifteen-year-long Duke study found that optimistic heart patients had a 30 percent higher chance of survival. Another fifteen-year study of three thousand heart disease sufferers showed that the optimistic patients lived 20 percent longer. Other studies say there's no difference. The evidence is especially weak linking optimism and recovery from cancer. Despite the claims of pop psychologists and books like *The Secret*, you can't think your way out of cancer with a positive attitude (more on that later).

Just as important, overoptimism is probably harmful. You have to be neurotic and realistic enough to go for regular checkups and take your meds. You need enough determination to attend to the details. A ninety-year longevity study by Howard Friedman, a University of California–Riverside psychology professor, found that a low but persistent level of worry about your health is correlated with longer lives.

So that's what I'll adopt: moderate optimism with a soupçon of anxiety. I can handle that.

As I leave, my grandfather plants his hands on the arms of his recliner and hoists himself up, over my protestations. He grabs Jane's shoulder to steady himself. He's bent over, his spine at a forty-five-degree angle to the ground, his legs wobbly. "We will see you soon?" he asks.

"Absolutely," I say.

Checkup: Month 4

Weight: 165

Miles walked writing this book thus far: 85 (My goal is to make this a thousand-mile book.)

Number of walnuts eaten this month: 790

Pounds lifted on squat machine (3 sets, 15 reps): 40

Glasses of goat's milk drunk: 10 (Many of the longest-lived civilizations drink goat's milk, according to *The Blue Zones*.)

Overall health: not good. I got a cold. Despite devoting most of my waking hours to being healthy, I got a cold.

Jennifer Ackerman's book *Ah-Choo!*, a history of colds, has a great quote about colds from the nineteenth-century poet Charles Lamb. "If you told me the world will be at an end tomorrow, I should just say, 'Will it?' . . . My skull is a Grub Street attic to let."

My skull is definitely atticlike. I can't find any coherent thoughts in there. But unlike Lamb, I'm more annoyed than apathetic. How could my body betray me?

Maybe I shouldn't be surprised. My immune system has always been overly welcoming of germs. It's far too polite, the biological equivalent of a southern hostess inviting y'all nice microbes to stay awhile and have some artichoke dip. I get a half-dozen colds per year. Julie, on the other hand, rarely gets sick. My kids should thank me for marrying up the immune system ladder.

For this cold, I've tried all the cures and treatments with any half-reliable evidence behind them. Zinc supplements, gargling with salt water, sleep, and using a neti pot. (All the others—echinacea, Airborne, megadoses of vitamin C, hot-water bottles on your head—have, sadly, little scientific support.)

The neti pot was the one that surprised me most. In case you've never seen it, it looks like a teapot, but instead of pouring raspberry zinger into a cup, you pour salt water into your nostril. The water gushes up to the sinus, splashes around a bit, then streams out the other nostril. The idea behind it is nasal irrigation, which thins the mucus, making it easier to expel.

It's a profoundly unnatural feeling, this meandering river inside your cranium. I coughed. I sputtered. I suppressed terror. I tilted my head in anatomically unsound angles. But in the end, it was far better than expected. It opened up my sinuses and cleared out the gunk. The inside of my head felt big and clear, a skull-size version of Montana. I plan to use my neti pot every day.

Julie used it, too. The next morning, not knowing what it was, she used it as a holder for Lucas's soft-boiled egg. I was horrified. She shrugged. Which brings me to . . .

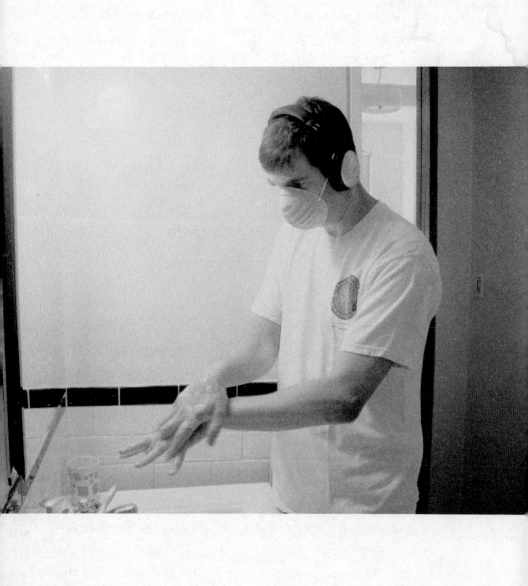

Chapter 5

The Immune System

The Quest to Conquer Germs

THANKS TO MY COLD, I've decided to devote this month to germs. It's a topic of great passion for me.

For years, I've been a huge consumer of germ porn. Perhaps you're familiar with the genre. I'm talking about those news segments that warn you that there are more germs on your remote control than on your toilet seat. Your sponge is a hot zone, and your wallet should be handled with a bio hazard suit.

The news will cut to footage of unwashed hands under black light, all Jackson Pollocked with glowing purple germ splotches.

I love the elaborate metaphors they use to convey the unimaginable number of germs. You have more germs in your gut right now than humans that ever lived on earth. (This is true.) If the germs on your hand were turned into drops of water, they'd fill an Olympic swimming pool (also true.) If the germs in your door handle were turned into letters on a page, the resulting document would be longer than the collected works of Joyce Carol Oates, and that includes her young adult fiction and boxing essays (probably true).

I love when they zoom in on a close-up on a particularly menacing-looking Aspergillus or a Clostridium. Check out those flagella! So titillating.

Germ porn probably isn't good for me, but it provides a perverse masochistic pleasure. It feeds into my germaphobia, a condition I've been struggling with for years, long before it became a familiar trope for TV detectives. (A couple of random examples: I prefer the air shake to the handshake. I don't like to clink wineglasses during a toast, unless I can clink the bottom of the glass, where the germ colonies are presumably sparser. And so on.)

Julie hates when I watch germ reports. She's on the opposite end of the spectrum. Our society is too hygiene obsessed, she says, and it's turning us into immunological pansies. Go ahead, she'll tell the boys, play in the sandbox, despite what Daddy says about residual fecal matter. Drink from that water fountain. A few months ago, Zane was eating an ice cream cone from the overpriced ice cream shop in our neighborhood. Then his scoop fell on the sidewalk. Amazingly, he didn't get upset. Instead, he got down on all fours and started licking it off the pavement like a golden retriever. A woman walking behind him gasped. "Oh my God." But Julie? She had no problem with it. New York is one big dinner plate.

Which is why she's even less happy about the visit I'm about to make. I am meeting with the Ron Jeremy of microbial fetish videos: Dr. Philip Tierno, the director of clinical microbiology and immunology at New York University Langone Medical Center. Also known as Dr. Germ. You might recognize Tierno from his segments on the *Today* show. The one on pillows featured millions of skin-eating dust mites, and has made me lose at least a week of sleep. He's the expert of experts.

"He's an enabler," Julie says. She might have a point.

But if my goal is to be the healthiest person alive, I've got to figure out the best way to conquer these germs.

I arrive at Tierno's midtown lab, where I find him studying a slide of toxic bacilli. He's bald, with a neat white beard and round wire-rim glasses. He sticks out his hand to greet me.

What? Dr. Germ wants to shake hands? That makes no sense at all. I respond by offering him my elbow for an elbow bump.

"Ah, this guy knows what he's doing," says Tierno. I beam. We go back to his cluttered office, filled with a microscope, eleven bottles of cleaning fluids, and two thousand biology books stacked in towering piles. Bach plays in the background.

First, Tierno wants me to know that germs suffer from some bad PR. Most bacteria are harmless. In fact, human beings are mostly germs. We are walking around with 90 percent germ cells, and just 10 percent human cells with our DNA. They're in our gut, in our mouth, in our eyebrows.

We came from germs. The oldest sign of life on earth is a fossilized germ cell found in Australia from 3.5 billion years ago.

"There are 156,000 categories of germs around, but only a small percentage are pathogenic. Maybe two thousand of these."

Ah, but those two thousand—you don't want them anywhere near you. Consider that infectious disease is still the leading cause of death in the world. Here's a disturbing statistic: Every year, a hundred thousand people in the world die because of infections they got *at the hospital* (they are called nosocomial infections). Another one: Every year, germs in food sicken an astounding 76 million people in the United States, according to the Centers for Disease Control.

Dr. Tierno started his road to germ whisperer when he was in eighth grade and read a biography of Louis Pasteur. I mention I'm a fan of Joseph Lister, the British surgeon who first developed the idea of sterile surgery.

"Semmelweis was an even bigger hero," says Tierno, of the Hungarian physician Ignaz Semmelweis. "He used to wash his hands after dealing with pregnant women, whereas most obstetricians just wiped their hands on their smocks, and killed by passing an infection from one woman to the other."

Hand washing is one of Dr. Tierno's passions. He thinks America needs a massive public education campaign on it, along the lines of our antismoking PR blitz. "It's the single most important thing you can do for your health," he says. "Eighty percent of all infections are transmitted by direct or indirect contact."

The key is to do it well, which few of us do. Most of us are hardly better than the French aristocrats in the court of Louis XIV. Back then, says Tierno, doctors advised washing only the tips of the fingers, for fear that water transmitted disease.

Tierno—who says he hasn't had a cold in four years—walks me down the hall to the bathroom for a hand-washing demo. He squirts the liquid soap onto his hands. He lathers up for forty-five seconds before even putting his hands under the water.

"In between the fingers. In between the nails."

He squishes and slides his hands together. He digs under his nails with his thumb and flicks his wrist. It's a virtuoso performance, like Yo-Yo Ma playing the cello or Al Pacino screaming obscenities. It's a long way from the average person's five-second dunk.

"Happy Birthday, Philly Boy," he sings as he finishes up. "Happy birthday to you." (For those who don't know, you're supposed to sing the entire birthday song during washing, to make sure you take your time.)

When we get back to his office, I grill him on the questions he gets from every John Q. Germaphobe:

Do Purell and other hand sanitizers work?

Yes. "You need to make sure you use enough. A quarter-size dollop." Studies show that it cuts the risk of colds by at least 40 percent.

"I love it, but my wife hates the smell," I tell him.

Dr. Tierno sniffs his hands. "What's to hate? Tell her it's like vodka."

Incidentally, I spent some time on the Purell website, where you can find a list of ninety-nine places germs lurk (in-flight magazines, movie tickets, gas-pump keypads, hotel room a/c controls, and on and on). It's hilarious and terrifying. The only place they don't mention is the Purell dispensers themselves. You know they're coated with germs. It's one of health's cruelest catch-22s.

Do Purell and antibacterial soap create supergerms? Like MRSA?

"No. Germs don't develop a resistance to alcohol or antibiotic soaps. They *can* develop a resistance to antibiotics." Tierno recommends against popping antibiotics every time you get a cold. But in Tierno's view, Purell and antibacterial soaps don't cause supergerms.

Should I use antibacterial soap?

"Ordinarily, you don't need antibacterial soap. You can get along with regular soap and warm water." The exception is when you're cooking foods, especially meat. He doesn't believe that triclosan, a controversial chemical in many antibacterial soaps, poses any danger (more on toxins later).

What about a face mask?

He wears them on planes. "One time I was going to France, and I had a lady coughing right in back of me. And I asked the stewardess to have her moved to another seat because she was very sick. And the stewardess said, 'The plane is full, I can't.' I didn't have my mask, and I caught a cold three days after that." He won't let that happen again.

As I leave, I give him a copy of my Bible book. He thanks me, though he admits he'll wipe it down before reading.

I walk out feeling both exhilarated and stressed out. Julie's right. He is an enabler.

The Hygiene Hypothesis

In the interest of equal time, I decide to look into those on Julie's side of the germ fence. Many scientists agree with her.

They've named their theory the Hygiene Hypothesis. The idea is that children in modern first-world countries aren't exposed to enough germs, a situation that throws off the development of the immune system. Our immune cells don't get the chance to learn to recognize and assassinate the bad guys. Our overly sanitized world could be responsible for the dramatic rise in allergies and asthma.

I call up an immunologist named Mary Ruebush, author of *Why Dirt is Good*, a rallying cry for the Hygiene Hypothesis.

"The pendulum has swung," she tells me. "The first few millennia of human evolution, there was no thought of cleanliness. Then, when we realized there's a link between cleanliness and health, we went overboard."

Like Tierno, she claims superior health. "I don't remember having a cold or a headache, and I have absolutely no standards of hygiene whatsoever."

I suppress my instinct to say that I'm glad this is a phone interview.

"My standard for hand washing is this: If they look dirty or smell bad, then I wash them," she says.

Like Tierno, she has her own scary story about a plane ride.

"I sat next to an eight-year-old child who was traveling by himself. He proceeded to wipe the seat, the armrest, and the tray table before he would sit down. I was horrified."

I tell her about how my son licked ice cream off the sidewalk. "Good for him," she says. "He is going to be a healthy adult."

When I get off the phone, I tell Julie about Ruebesh's thesis. "That's a wise woman," Julie says.

Later that night, when Julie drops a cucumber slice on the floor, she bends down to pick it up and put it on Zane's plate.

"Hygiene Hypothesis!" she says gleefully. It's her new catchphrase.

I decide to spend a week implementing Tierno's Germ Battle Plan on myself. I promise Julie I'll leave her and the kids out of it.

In his book *The Secret Life of Germs*, Tierno gives a list of antiseptic-living suggestions, which I've transcribed onto my computer. On a Wednesday morning, I begin to implement them. Here's a small sample:

- Wipe down the phones and remote controls weekly. (Does wiping them with a moist paper towel really get the germs off? I wish I could boil my electronic equipment.)
- Soak all produce for five to ten minutes in a solution of water, hydrogen peroxide, and vinegar. ("Hydrogen peroxide?" asks our babysitter as I pour some into a bowl of apples. "Is that safe? I thought that's what you use to dye hair." It's in the book, I tell her.)
- Wash underwear separately from other clothes to prevent a transfer of fecal residue.

- Dry laundry in the sun, because the UV radiation kills germs (a clothesline doesn't work in New York, so I lay my shirts on the outside part of the air conditioner).
- Remove showerheads and clean them with a wire brush to root out legionella, the cause of Legionnaires' disease (still have to do this).
- Vacuum curtains and upholstery regularly.
- Zap damp sponges in the microwave for one or two minutes.
- Put hypoallergenic sheets and pillowcases on your bed to keep the dust mites from snacking on your dead skin flakes, because dust mites can cause allergies. (The ones I bought are kind of slippery, but they make me feel better. Tierno himself takes his germproof sheets with him when he goes to a hotel. I put that on my to-do list.)

It's been half a day, and I'm not even close to finishing my list. Germ warfare is a full-time job. Though I do notice something strange. Aside from being busy, I have another feeling: righteousness.

Maybe it's my imagination, but now I crave more order in every part of my life. I'm more annoyed when Julie's late to dinner. I'm more concerned when my son Jasper hangs around with the rambunctious elements in his class.

Does my punctiliousness have anything to do with my germ obsession? Perhaps not. But the brain is an odd place, and it's possible that germaphobia has colored my moral view. I read a fascinating *New York Times* op-ed by two scientists who argue that the more obsessed you are with germs, the more politically conservative you become.

They conducted an experiment in which they asked subjects

about their "moral, social and fiscal" attitudes. "Merely standing near a hand-sanitizing dispenser led people to report more conservative political beliefs," they write. "Apparently, the slightest signal that germs might be present is enough to shift political attitudes toward the right."

The professors—Peter Liberman at Queens College and David Pizarro at Cornell—offer the explanation that early humans often came into contact with other tribes that harbored dangerous germs. So humans evolved to have a feeling of disgust at The Other, which helped keep interactions to a minimum. This sense of disgust is correlated to conservative, more wary-of-foreigners worldview.

When I told one of my token conservative friends this theory, he said it sounded absurd. But, he added, at least it gave him license to call liberals dirty.

Checkup: Month 5

Weight: 164

Push-ups till exhaustion: 26

Dollars spent at GNC on supplements that have iffy scientific
support (e.g., açaí berry, resveratrol): $127

Avocados consumed: 1.5 per day

The big breaking news for this month is: My gym sessions are altering my body. My chest has a little curve to it, like a very gentle slope on a putting green. When I went running the other day, I could feel my pecs bounce. This experience is new and curiously exhilarating.

I'm spending an embarrassing amount of time every night studying my torso in the mirror, trying to discern the progress. I have fantasies about running into Vlad the caveman and hearing him say, "I'm sorry for those comments about your chest. Boy, how wrong I was!"

I now understand why all these reality-show stars walk around with their shirts off. If you spend that much time sculpting your body, you want to display your work of art. Otherwise, it's like keeping a Gauguin in the garage under a sheet.

I've started to notice other men's bodies as well. I have biceps envy. I look for their veins in their arms and compare them to mine. Never before have I cared about having visible blood vessels.

Or maybe I did. Looking back, I don't think I admitted to myself how much I've been self-conscious about my concave chest for years. I pretended not to care. I pretended I was above such concerns. But I also hated changing in the locker room, and would keep my T-shirt on at the beach.

My new hint of muscle makes me crave more. At the suggestion of my friend Tim Ferriss—author of *The 4-Hour Body*—I'm taking daily doses of the supplement creatine, an acid found in skeletal muscle.

At the same time, I'm aware that this obsession with size is ridiculous. There's only a mild correlation between what we consider healthy *looking*, and *being* healthy—especially when it comes to muscle definition. Do the Okinawans in Japan—the longest-lived people on earth—have six-packs abs? I doubt it. Not in the pictures I've seen.

On the food front, I'm still working on my portion control. Before each meal, I say my 80 percent prayer (this is from the Japanese proverb that you should only eat until you are four-fifths full). I'm observing my chewdaism. I'm addicted to these diabolical dried mangoes, so, at the suggestion of social psychologist Sam Sommers from Tufts University, I've repackaged them into a bunch of tiny Ziploc bags—one mango slice per bag. It actually works. My mind thinks that it's getting a full portion, even if the portion is one slice. My mind, in other words, is an idiot.

But despite my limited victories with portion control, I keep coming back to the fundamental question: What the heck should I put in those portions? What should I eat? Which of America's ten thousand experts should I listen to? I pledge to make answering this question my next month's mission.

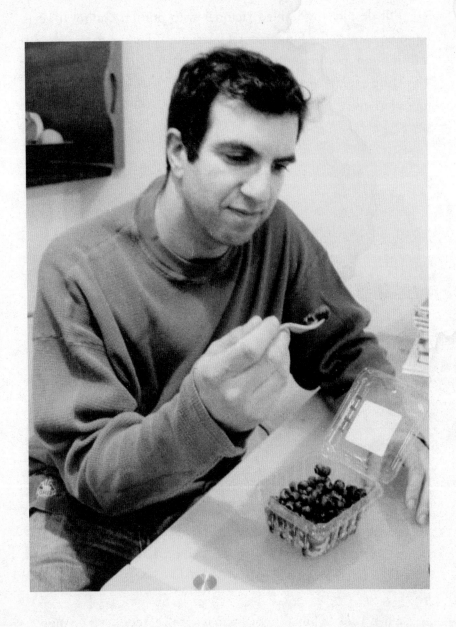

Chapter 6

The Stomach, Revisited

The Quest for the Perfect Meal

A FEW DAYS AGO, I stumbled across what sounded like an interesting perspective: a Colorado-based doctor named Steven Bratman who has discovered what he calls a new eating disorder: "orthorexia nervosa." He defines "orthorexia" as an unhealthy obsession with healthy foods.

The idea is that if you are unduly fixated on eating healthily, you'll stress yourself out—so much so that the damage from the stress outweighs any potential benefits of the good food. It's an intriguing idea, so I e-mail Bratman to request an interview.

He agrees, responding that he has "a number of salty comments."

Salty. Interesting choice. He even uses unhealthy foods as adjectives.

When I talk to him, Dr. Bratman is as full of sodium as promised. He says the obsession with healthy food is "stupid." Its practitioners are filled with "hot air." In the end, too much emphasis on your diet is harmful because "you don't have balance in your life."

Once upon a time, Bratman himself had a fetish for healthy food. Back in the seventies, he was an organic farmer and chef at a commune in upstate New York. He spent his days steaming tomatoes and arguing about whether aluminum pots were poisonous. He reached a breaking point when, he says, "a particularly enthusiastic visitor tried to convince me that slicing a vegetable would destroy its energy field." In frustration, Bratman chased the guy away with a flat Chinese cleaver.

After his fall from heath food grace, he coined the term "orthorexia." The "ortho" part derives from the Greek for "correct," and the "rexia" is from the word for "appetite." Hence orthorexia, the mania for the correct diet. The condition hasn't yet made it into *The Diagnostic and Statistical Manual of Mental Disorders*, the Bible of psychological illnesses. But it's gained some fans among therapists and researchers. Bratman wrote a book about the condition called *Health Food Junkies*.

The symptoms include:

- When you stray from healthy food, you're filled with guilt and self-loathing.
- You become socially isolated because it's hard to eat at the same table as less conscientious friends.
- Healthy eating has become your replacement religion, making you feel virtuous. You regard omnivores with disgust.

In Bratman's words, "a day filled with wheatgrass juice, tofu and quinoa biscuits may come to feel as holy as one spent serving the destitute and homeless."

So according to Bratman, health food fetishism will hurt me. It's an intriguing idea. But even if it's true, I need some basic instructions on what to eat to be the healthiest person alive. What does he recommend?

"Don't get fat and get your vitamins."

That's it? That's his health advice? I press him for more.

Bratman resists. The problem is, everyone wants secrets: *Selenium will prevent bladder cancer, so eat Brazil nuts! Flavonoids prevent heart disease, so eat pineapple!* But the science just isn't there yet. He tells me all health advice can be boiled down to a single paragraph:

"Eating fruits and vegetables is vaguely logical. Get sleep. Don't live in the most polluted parts of the world. Don't smoke. Don't do unsafe things like skiing and hang gliding, which are inconceivably more dangerous than eating 'unhealthy' foods. Exercise is pretty likely good for you. Don't drink too much alcohol—one or two drinks a day. And that's about it."

In Bratman's view, all the hype about antioxidants and glycemic indices are unproven. Nutrition science is barely more evidence based than phrenology. Or as Bratman puts it, "hardly better than college bullshitting."

This stance has not made him friends in the health food community. His website has a section devoted to reader hate mail. One of the milder samples: "Dr. Bratman, you are a moron. Please go to Mickey Dee's and chow down on a few Big Macs and don't call me in the morning. I guess Monsanto's GMO products, high fructose corn syrup, aspartame, processed sugar and flour are great for us . . . Have a great day and don't forget to supersize, you idiot."

I don't think Bratman is an idiot. Mind you, I don't agree with him. His conclusions are far too radical for me. But I believe he provides an important cautionary voice. Because the more I learn, the more I realize we know a lot less about nutrition than the newspaper headlines would have you believe. Food is frustratingly complicated. It resists reductionism. Often, we'll identify what we think is a secret healthy ingredient—carrots have beta carotene, which is why they prevent cancer. So we'll give people beta-carotene supplements, only to find out it's not so simple. Beta-carotene supplements *increased* the instances of lung cancer among smokers in a large study in Finland.

Your everyday carrot is filled with so many micronutrients, we don't yet know how they interact with one another. Michael Pollan, author of *The Omnivore's Dilemma*, likes to say, "Nutrition science is where surgery was in the 16th century. It's interesting. But would you really want them operating on you?" The best we can do, to paraphrase Pollan, is to eat whole foods, mostly plants, and not too much.

Ben Goldacre—a British doctor, skeptic, and author of the book *Bad Science*—is even harsher. He talks about nutritionists' lack of "intellectual horsepower" and their "crimes" against sensible dietary advice.

The problem is, it's hard to conduct randomized placebo-controlled studies on humans and their diets. If you could lock ten thousand people in identical rooms for eighty years and feed half of them nothing but vegan food and feed the other half nothing but steak and eggs, and keep everything else the same, you could have some real data. But unless a Bond villain decides to pursue a doctorate in nutrition, that's not going to happen.

Instead, much of our nutrition knowledge comes from two sources. First, animal studies. Which can be enlightening, but don't always translate to humans.

And second, epidemiological studies. I'm vastly oversimplifying here, but an epidemiological study is when scientists analyze statistics in a population to determine the cause of a disease. It's a hugely useful tool. Epidemiology helped link tobacco and lung cancer, and cholera and dirty water. But it's also got limitations, especially when it comes to something as complicated as food and drink. There are hundreds of confounding factors that can throw off the results.

Consider alcohol. The data show that drinking is healthy because moderate drinkers live longer than teetotalers. But what if it's not the drinking, but the social interaction that goes along with drinking? What if parties and sporting events are healthy, not vodka?

The science journalist Gary Taubes wrote a great *New York Times Magazine* story on the problem, and sums it up this way: We often confuse correlation and causation. To quote a famous example: Diabetes rates are much lower in areas where people own passports. Therefore, you might conclude that owning a passport prevents diabetes. Right? Wrong. It's more likely that passport owners are wealthier, and wealthier people can afford healthier food.

These complexities make me feel both better and worse. Better because I now understand why nutrition headlines contradict each other every week. (Soy is the secret! Soy is poison!) It's not always out of stupidity or conspiracy. Sometimes it's just because it's so darn complicated.

But it's also dispiriting, because at least for now, there are no black-and-white answers.

The Battle for the Plate

That said, I can't give up. I still want to figure out some basic guidelines on what to eat.

First, let me start with what almost everyone agrees on, not counting Bratman. Study after study suggests we should be eating more whole foods, not processed foods—broccoli instead of french fries. We've got way too much sugar in our diet. And to a lesser extent, too much salt. And, as I mentioned before, we eat too much damn food.

In other words, almost everyone agrees our nation's typical fried and sugar-laden daily intake is a disaster. My aunt Marti calls it by the delightfully descriptive acronym SAD—Standard American Diet.

So there's a lot we all agree on. But there's also a lot of room for dispute. And man, is there dispute. The nutrition field resembles Congress. There are two warring tribes, and most everyone falls somewhere along the spectrum.

On the far left side, many advocate for the plant-based diet. On the far right, many argue for the low-carb, high-protein diet.

Currently, the advocates of the mostly plant diet have the majority. The holy text of radical plant fans is the bestselling 2005 book *The China Study* by T. Colin Campbell, a nutritional biochemistry professor at Cornell. It's an impressive book based on a huge twenty-year study of 880 million people in China. The conclusion? Eating animal products causes a large number of health problems, including heart disease, diabetes, breast cancer, macular degeneration, bowel cancer, osteoporosis, and others. The healthiest diet is one with no animal products at all, no beef, no poultry, no eggs, no fish, and no milk. Campbell doesn't like to call the diet "vegan," since that carries political tones. But essentially, it's vegan. So that's one side.

The other side is best represented by the aforementioned Gary Taubes, a brilliant journalist who wrote the books *Good Calories, Bad Calories* and *Why We Get Fat*. One of his big theses is that the low-fat diet is a sham. It's based on faulty science. In fact, America adopted the low-fat diet in the 1970s. That's the exact same era when the obesity epidemic began. The low-fat diet, he argues, has been a giant belly flop.

The real culprit isn't fat. It's carbohydrates—especially refined carbs. Here's Taubes: "Insulin puts fat in fat cells. That's what it does. And our insulin levels, for the most part, are determined by the carb-content of our diet—the quantity and quality of the carbohydrates consumed." The more concentrated the sugar in our carbs, the more dangerous they are.

Taubes and his camp recommend restricting carbs as much as possible, especially processed carbs, high-glycemic carbs (like bananas), and starchy carbs (like potatoes). Instead, they recommend eating more protein and good fats. They eat a lot of lean beef, eggs, fish, and all sorts of vegetables (spinach and broccoli, for instance). But little grain.

I'll tell you where I've stood for the last decade or so: On the spectrum, I've leaned more toward *The China Study* side. I'm not vegan. I still eat eggs and salmon. But I don't eat beef, pork, or lamb. I used to call myself a quasi-vegetarian. Now I prefer the trendier term "flexitarian."

There are two reasons I lean this way.

The first is because I'm biased. My lovable, eccentric aunt Marti has been drilling antimeat information into my brain since I was a kid.

She's showed me videos of the horrors of slaughterhouses. She's told me about each and every carcinogen allegedly found in meat. She'll make animal products as unappetizing as possible. If I'm eating ice cream, she'll say, "Are you enjoying your mucus? Because that's what ice cream is, essentially. Congealed mucus."

Her passion is hard to forget. I still remember one dinner at my grandfather's house. The whole extended family was there, and

Marti, at the time, refused to eat at the same table where flesh was being served. Half the family was fine with that. But the other half wanted chicken. The solution? We had to set up two separate tables in the dining room—a meat table and a nonmeat table. My diplomatic grandparents didn't want to take sides, so they sat at a *third* table in the middle, a dietary DMZ.

The second reason I opt for the plant-based diet is that, in technical matters, I tend to accept the beliefs of most scientists.

This semiblind acceptance is an unfortunate result of the arcanization of scientific knowledge. If I lived in the nineteenth century, I could judge for myself whether I thought Mendel's study on peas made sense. But can I judge whether C-reactive protein is a better predictor of heart disease than LDL levels? Not without devoting several months of my life to that single question. It's why I believe in global warming. If a survey by the National Academy of Sciences finds that 97 percent of climate scientists believe in man-made climate change, I feel it's wise to accept their view.

This stance has its downsides. Science isn't perfect, and suffers from biases, fads and fraud. But the upsides far outweigh the dangers.

And right now the majority of scientists advocate a diet with lots of plants and reduced animal-based fats and protein. Even the USDA's 2011 dietary guidelines inch toward the plant-based side. In the past, some nutritionists slammed the USDA Food Pyramid for being too heavily influenced by the pro-meat agriculture lobby. But the latest version took the step of recommending minimal animal protein. You can see it in the 2011 MyPlate, in which protein makes up just 20 percent of the ideal meal, with beans strongly recommended.

But I don't ignore Taubes's advice. He makes a persuasive case against simple carbs, one that has altered what I put in my mouth.

I'm now loath to put anything white in my mouth, not counting cauliflower and straws (the latter of which may help cut down on corrosion to the teeth, especially if they are placed in the back of the tongue).

Shopping the Perimeters

To help me figure out the healthiest diet, I decide I need a guided tour of the grocery. I called Marion Nestle, a professor at New York University, author of *What to Eat*, and a highly respected thinker in all things nutritional. She met me at Whole Foods in midtown New York.

I chose Whole Foods not just because it's got lots of healthy food. But also because it's got lots of *unhealthy* food disguised as healthy food. Sugar and fat in antioxidant clothing. And I'm a sucker for faux health food.

It's been a significant portion of my diet for the past decade. I eat sweetened granola bars and organic cereal that tastes like off-brand versions of Frosted Flakes. An embarrassing confession: I used to drink VitaminWater. Look at that, I said to myself, it's got green tea extract! If I'd been around in the nineteenth century, I'd be the first to say, Yes, Mr. Barnum, I *would* like to see the egress. Sounds fascinating.

I'm aware on some level VitaminWater is gussied-up sugar water—a bottle contains 32.5 grams of sugar, nearly as much as a can of Coca-Cola Classic's 39 grams. But I still like eating and drinking this ersatz health food. It gives me a virtuous feeling, even if that virtue is unfounded. At least I'm doing something, you know? And it says "Healthy" right there on the package.

I meet Nestle—whose name, incidently, is pronounced NESS-el, not like the tollhouse cookie makers—at the bottom of the escalator. She's with her boyfriend, Mal Nesheim, a brilliant (and farm-raised) Cornell University nutrition professor.

Nestle wants to make it clear she's pro–Whole Foods, despite its flaws. She regrets mentioning its nickname "Whole Paycheck" in her book. "That was trite," she says. Yes, it can gobble up your bank account, but the fact that healthy food costs more than artery-clogging food shouldn't be dismissed with a glib phrase. It's a complicated issue. (For one thing, Americans spend much less of their paycheck on food than Europeans—an estimated 10 percent to 30 percent. We might have to adjust our priorities.)

I ask her to show me the least healthy food in Whole Foods. "Oh, let's go look at the breakfast cereals. They're always the most fun."

We walk to aisle eight. And there, we find box after box of cereal with pictures of farmhouses and grain fields. She picks up a box. She slides her glasses from atop her curly gray hair to her nose, and lasers in on the nutrition label. Nestle has spent more time reading nutrition labels than most Americans have spent reading novels (which, I suppose, isn't saying much). And she knows how to unlock their secrets.

"Evaporated cane juice," she reads aloud. "Translation: sugar." Really? It sounds so natural.

"Organic molasses," she keeps reading. "Translation: sugar." It's not better?

"It's got a few nutrients. But not enough to make a difference. Sugar is sugar."

What about agave nectar? That's the healthy sugar, right? "No."

Some sugars are slightly better than others, but only slightly. If you eat too much, they all end up as fat and can lead to metabolic syndrome and diabetes and all sorts of other horrible maladies.

A little farther down the aisle are all the faux-healthy protein bars. "Oh, look, it's organic!" says Nestle, with more than a bit of sarcasm. "There's now research that shows that when people see the word 'organic,' they think it has fewer calories."

So if high-cane-juice cereals are the least healthy, what foods are the healthiest? Nestle leads me to the produce section.

"Here. Anything in here."

"Blueberries?" I say. "They're a superfood."

"Yes, they're healthy," says Nestle. "But I don't believe in super-foods."

Hold on now. What's this?

Nestle thinks that we have an outsize obsession with ranking our fruits and vegetables. Her argument is, in a way, similar to Bratman's. Our reasoning is too reductive. We figure: Fruits and vegetables are good for you. Fruits and vegetables have antioxidants. Therefore it's the antioxidants in the fruits and vegetables that are good for you.

This type of thinking leads us to believe idea that the fruit with the most antioxidants is the best. It makes us overlook all the non-superfoods—what one writer called "Clark Kent" foods—such as apples and oranges, which are perfectly healthy. Antioxidants are just one of dozens of good chemicals in food.

Nestle says that the blueberry obsession can be traced, in part, to the brilliant marketing efforts of the Maine wild blueberry growers. A decade ago, the Maine blueberry industry was in trouble. In years past, they'd tried several strategies: They attempted to market blueberries as candy. Even odder, they ran a campaign suggesting blueberries as a condiment to put on hamburgers. Nothing worked. But when a Tufts study said that wild blueberries had a high antioxidant rating, they ran with it, and blueberries have become the prototypical health food.

We finished our Whole Foods adventure and went to lunch at a nearby café. I ordered the Bibb lettuce salad, dressing on the side.

The waitress looked at Nestle and Nesheim. "Are the profiteroles good?" asks Nestle.

"So good," says the waitress.

"I'll have that."

Huh. I'm here with quite possibly the most knowledgeable nutritionist in the world, and she's having a plateful of sugar and fat.

"You've got to enjoy food," says Nestle, noticing my raised eyebrows. "It's one of the great things in life." She assures me that she eats plenty of fruits and veggies as well.

I'm not a doctor, but I can say with certainty: Marion Nestle does not have orthorexia.

Checkup: Month 6

Weight: 160
Average number of errands sprinted per day: 3
Waist size: 34 (down from 35)
Pounds lifted on squat machine: 90 (improvement!)
Sleep per night: 6.4 hours
Half-ounce Purell bottles used this month: 14

Overall state: I'm feeling okay, though a little stressed out about how much of my book advance I'm spending on fitness equipment. My closets are filling up with a bizarre collection of weights, gadgets, and clothes. It's as if I was given access to a SkyMall catalog, a cell phone, and a jug of whiskey.

I am now the proud owner of a yoga mat and a swiss exercise ball. I also have a compression suit from Under Armour. This skintight silver outfit is supposed to help your muscles recover more quickly postworkout by directing blood flow. I wore it to the gym one day, and got plenty of feedback from the gym staff. "Hey, Superman!" "Nanu, nanu!" And so on. But there's something comforting and womblike about its snugness.

I own a custom-fitted mouthpiece that is supposedly similar to the one worn by Derek Jeter. A modern spin on my eight-grade retainer, the mouthpiece is designed to open your airways, and relax you by unclenching your jaw. It does make running easier—though I can get the same effect for free by jutting my jaw forward a half inch while running.

Of all the gadgets that clutter my closet, the most successful has been one of the simplest: a twenty-dollar pedometer. Actually, I have two, since Julie agreed to join me in my pedometer experiment.

Studies show that the more you pay attention to your body's statistics, the greater the chance you'll adopt a healthy lifestyle. This idea underpins the Quantified Self movement, in which adherents track everything from caloric output to selenium levels.

The mere act of weighing yourself daily makes it more likely you'll shed pounds, according to a University of Minnesota study. Keeping a food journal makes you eat fewer fatty foods, according to another study. And pedometers make you walk more.

Julie and I wear our silver bubble-shaped pedometers clipped to our pants. Our stated goal is to rack up ten thousand steps per day—the amount recommended by the American Heart Association.

The pedometer doesn't just spur us to move, though it certainly does that. It changes the way we *think* about movement. What was once a chore becomes a game. The other day, I spent half an hour looking for Lucas's missing stuffed elephant. Normally, that would be half an hour of frustration and snarling. Instead, I focused on the fact that I notched five hundred steps. Give me more missing stuffed animals! You got any keys I can search for? I'll take anything on.

My treadmill desk gets me past the ten-thousand mark most days. But Julie doesn't go down without a fight. She marches in place while making coffee or talking on the phone.

We were walking to the park the other day, and I noticed that she was taking quick, tiny, ballerina-size steps. "I've got shorter legs than you," she said. "I've got to play to my strengths."

She's enjoying the competition. We're getting along so well, I figure I'll devote the next month to another joint activity.

Chapter 7

The Genitals

The Quest to Have More Sex

IT'S A DEBATE THAT'S BEEN around almost as long as sex itself: Is the act of intercourse healthy for you? Or will it kill you?

Weighing in on the "sex is dangerous" side were, naturally, Victorian-era experts. Not all Victorians lived up to their repressive stereotype, but others did so with enthusiasm. One of my favorite characters from the encyclopedia was the chastity-obsessed nine-teenth-century health guru Sylvester Graham. Graham disapproved of lust and sex in general, with masturbation as his white whale. Touching yourself, he argued, leads inexorably to insanity, weakness, and death.

His prescription? Logically enough, bland foods. He believed the key to lowering the nefarious sex drive was a tasteless, spiceless diet. Which is how Graham came to invent one of the first health foods: the graham cracker, a snack that was originally made with

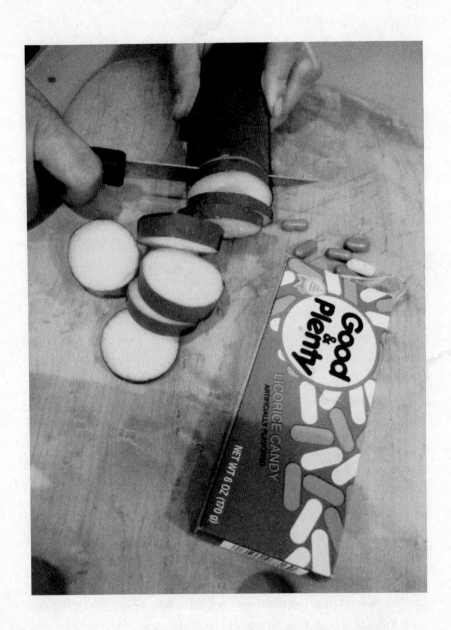

wheat germ, wheat bran and a little honey and was intended to quell the passions in hormonal adolescent boys. (I can't speak for the original, but the modern bran-free version doesn't seem to work so well in this regard. At least based on the following anecdotal evidence: I ate a lot of s'mores in high school.)

Graham was on the extreme end, but he represents a prevalent strain of sexaphobic thinking. A friend gave me a 1901 book called *What a Man of Forty-five Ought to Know*. It was a gag gift (I'm approaching forty-five, though not there yet), but it was a fascinating read. The book soberly warns that middle-aged men will "find that the act of coition is generally followed by a period of lassitude or weariness more pronounced and more prolonged than anything he has previously experienced. Nature is thus sounding her warnings and admonishing the individual of the importance of the utmost care in the use of a secretion which can now ill be spared, and which is of utmost importance in vitalizing every department of the physical economy." I'm pretty sure this means stop humping.

On the other hand, history is filled with experts who argued sex is a key to robust health. The Taoists in the eleventh century believed sex resulted in the joining of the Energy, and could even result in immortality—especially if the men didn't ejaculate. Frankly, that seems a high price.

Other experts have said it's dangerous *not* to have an orgasm, especially for women. Physicians from the time of the ancient Greeks right on up to the 1950s believed that noxious fluids built up inside unmarried women, causing "hysteria." The solution was a vigorous between-the-legs massage. In fact, as Mary Roach points out in her excellent book *Bonk: The Curious Coupling of Science and Sex*, the earliest vibrators were sold not to women, but to doctors to help relieve them of their manual labor.

Also on the pro-sex side: noted medical theorist Ernest Borgnine.

I was watching the ninety-four-year-old *Poseiden Adventure* actor on a morning talk show, and the host asked him the secret to his long life. He replied: "I masturbate a lot." So there you go. QED.

Recent science has come down on the side of sex as healthy. For the most part, that is. It has to be the right kind of sex: consensual, of course. And not so acrobatic that it results in broken body parts (penis fractures occur in about a thousand energetic men a year in the United States). And if you're out of shape, there's a slightly higher risk of heart attack in the hours after sex.

But overall, frequent orgasms have multiple health benefits. Among them, according to Rutgers University researchers: lower stress, and decreased rates of heart disease, breast cancer, and endometriosis. A study in the *Journal of the American Medical Association* found that men who ejaculated twenty-one or more times a month had a lower prostate cancer risk.

Also longevity. One British study concluded that two or more orgasms per week cut your risk of dying from heart disease in half. Another claims that Protestant ministers live longer than Catholic priests. Of course, it's always best to take epidemiological studies like this with a grain of Himalayan crystal salt. (Also, no disrespect to Dr. Borgnine, but most of the data out there is about two-person sex.)

Sex almost certainly helps a relationship. When you have an orgasm, your brain pumps out the attachment chemical oxytocin, heightening feelings of closeness. In fact, semen itself contains oxytocin, which helps boost feelings of postcoital intimacy.

Oh, and don't forget about curing hiccups. In *Bonk*, Roach cites a report in the journal *Canadian Family Physician* called "Sexual Intercourse as a Potential Treatment for Intractable Hiccups." It was a case study of an Israeli man whose four-day hiccup spree vanished after sex with his wife.

And if that's not enough, sex is just plain good exercise. There have been a handful—not a lot—of studies on the aerobic benefits of bedroom behavior. In one study, ten married couples tested out different positions. It wasn't the most romantic of settings, unless you happen to be a fan of Mistress Roxy's Dungeon Club. The husbands were covered with electrodes and kiss-preventing face masks to measure their breathing rates. Regardless, the conclusion was that, yes, sex does provide moderate exercise, and that the man-on-top missionary position burned the most calories for men. (The women's exertions, unfairly enough, went unmeasured.)

Which brings me to the practical question: In terms of optimum health, how often should I be engaging in said horizontal workout? I asked Dr. Debra Herbenick of the Kinsey Institute. She said it's hard to say. There's no scientific consensus.

But it does seem that this is one area where more is almost surely better, at least up to a point.

Julie doesn't want me saying exactly how often we have sex. That is probably just as well. But she will let me say that it's somewhere below the U.S. average, which, according to a 2001 survey, is 132 times per year. However, it's above the Japanese average, which is 37 times per year. (And yet Japan has a high percentage of centenarians, so an idle libido isn't necessarily a death sentence.)

Early on in this project, I proposed an every-night schedule for the book, a Hail mary that, frankly, neither of us wanted. So that went nowhere. But for the sake of health, I should at least try to nudge us up to the putative U.S. average.

So on a Thursday night, I start Project Libido.

I've been researching aphrodisiacs in an effort to enlist some chemical help. So I've prepared a romantic meal for our special night:

Brazil nuts
celery and peanut butter
red ginseng
asparagus
walnuts

All are alleged to boost the sex drive, some with bioflavonoids to open up the blood vessels, others that raise testosterone, and still others that mimic pheromones.

I laid them all out on a tray and brought them to Julie while she was watching *Mad Men*. A devoted wife, Julie took a bite out of each one, save the peanut butter (she hates it). She continues watching *Mad Men*. It's been ten minutes, and so far she hasn't ripped off her bra and jumped on top of me.

After the show, we go to the bedroom. I've brought a water mister and I spritz the air in our bedroom with a special concoction.

"What's in that?" asked Julie.

"This scent causes the biggest increase in blood flow to women's privates, according to one study."

Julie sniffs the air. "I can't place it."

"Good and Plenty and cucumber," I say.

Earlier, I'd soaked five pieces of the candy and three slices of cucumber in a glass of water, then poured it into the sprayer.

"Someone actually tested that? Good and Plenty and cucumber? That's the combination they came up with?" she asks.

"That's what the science says."

"What about Mike and Ike and turnips?"

"It's under review."

She's not annoyed, just incredulous. Unfortunately, Julie might be right to be a little skeptical. When I later asked Rockefeller

University odor researcher Leslie Vosshall about it, she said, "Ah, the famous Good and Plenty study. Well, it hasn't been replicated. It's not one of the most pressing issues in biomedical research."

Here's the sad news. Almost all existing aphrodisiacs are scientifically dubious. There's a whiff of evidence that daily ingestion of red ginseng can boost libido a bit. One meta-analysis says that maca powder and saffron might also be effective. But overall, science hasn't yet cracked the code. They may soon. But not yet. Earlier this week, I'd e-mailed Dr. Helen Fisher for aphrodisiac advice. Fisher is a Rutgers professor, the author of *Why We Love: The Nature and Chemistry of Romantic Love*, and the expert on this topic. She wrote me back:

> There are only a couple true aphrodisiacs: testosterone, and perhaps dopamine.
>
> There is no evidence at all that any particular food or liquor stimulates sex drive. But testosterone does. This is the hormone of sexual desire. And these days, it is available by injection, patch, or cream.
>
> Doctors often prescribe a dopamine agonist instead though. Dopamine [a neurochemical associated with pleasure] does seem to stimulate sexual desire, but not directly. It probably does it by triggering the activity of testosterone, as these two chemical systems tend to stimulate each other.
>
> So if you are really thinking of a "natural aphrodisiac," go do something thrilling together. Novelty, danger, and excitement all drive up dopamine in the brain.
>
> So skip the food and take a vacation together to somewhere new. The novelty will do what oysters and peanut butter never will.

A vacation isn't on the horizon right now, not with the kids anchoring us to the apartment. So my brainstorm? Julie loves roller coasters. Roller coasters are exciting. The iPhone has a remarkably lifelike roller-coaster game.

When I show her the iPhone app, Julie gives me a look that says, and I'm paraphrasing here, "I appreciate the thought, but that's not going to work, so you can put it away now." I put it away.

"Okay, then. Let's go burn some calories," I tell Julie.

I know. Not exactly the eighteenth sonnet.

But I wanted to remind Julie that sex can be legitimate exercise. I even had the data to back it up. Two weeks ago, I bought a gadget called a Fitbit—a black, french-fry-size, motion-sensor device you clip to your waistband. It links to the Internet and keeps track of calories you expend.

To help with the calculations, Fitbit's website has a list of activities along with the estimated calories burned per hour. It's a long list. We're not just talking about walking, running, and jumping rope. They've listed any activity you can think of.

Vacuuming? That's 238 calories per hour.

Shuffleboard? 204 calories.

Cooking Indian bread on an outside stove? Also 204 calories per hour.

I show the printout to Julie, as we sit on the bed. She reads:

Sexual activity—passive, light effort, kissing, hugging—68 calories.

Sexual activity—general, moderate effort—88.

Sexual activity—active, vigorous effort—102 calories per
hour.

"Moderate effort sounds good," says Julie.

I agree. We're not vigorous-effort types anymore.

Besides, she points out, if we want a workout afterward, we can
always groom a horse (408 calories an hour).

I won't go into detail about our exercise session, but suffice it to
say, we fell pretty far short of the hour mark. So depending on how
much you believe Fitbit's stats—which, frankly, seem a tad low to
me—we didn't break 88 calories.

Even sadder: The following month—despite the big plans and
the dopamine and the scent of Good & Plenty—Julie and I fell
back into our old subaverage schedule. We're just not motivated
enough. I pledge to seek professional help. Before the end of the
project, I plan to see a urologist.

Checkup: Month 7

Weight: 158
Blood pressure: 110/70
Cans of steel-cut oatmeal consumed this year: 11
Average hours per day wearing noise-canceling earphones: 10
Pounds lifted on squat machine (15 reps): 150

To paraphrase James Brown, I feel moderately good. Every day,
I look at the digitally aged photo of myself and try to honor Old A.J.
I'm eating a little better. The cravings for sugar and salt still wash
over me, but they're weakening. (And because I've weaned myself
from salt, my palate has changed. It's more sensitive. When I break

down and have a potato chip, the saltiness is overwhelming, as if I'm emptying a shaker on my tongue.)

At the gym, Tony tries to work me hard enough to make my glasses steam up. "That was a lens fogger," he'll say proudly, after a set of fifty squats.

I'm trying, with moderate success, to control my stress. So I'm self-massaging every day. That is not a euphemism. Studies show that rubbing your own shoulders decreases levels of the stress hormone cortisol. So I rub myself while riding the bus or reading the paper.

My family, though, is becoming impatient with the project. My sons are annoyed that I won't eat cupcakes with them at birthday parties, opting instead for a plastic bag of carrots. They keep asking me why it's so important to me that I be healthy.

"It's so I don't get sick," I tell them one day as I spoon my steel-cut oatmeal. "So I can stay around and be with you for a long, long time."

"So you don't die?" says Lucas.

"Right. So I don't die."

I had been avoiding the D-word. But the kids cut right to it. My boys are well aware of death. My twins finish every story they make up with the same phrase: "Then everyone died. The end."

It works no matter the subject. "And the octopus went to the circus. He saw the lions and tigers and had some cotton candy. Then everyone died. The end." Or else, "Curious George climbed up the tree to get his kite. He got his kite. Then everyone died. The end."

I don't think they are being macabre. They are just looking for a tidy way to wrap up a complicated plot. It's effective, if a tad deus ex machina.

At the same time, they are starting to get concerned about this notion of death.

A few days ago, Lucas told me, "When I grow up, I want to be a character in a book so that I never die." That broke my heart, and made me want to warn him to avoid his own stories.

Around the same time, Zane begged me to put him on my shoulders so he could touch the ceiling in every room of our apartment. I told him I couldn't do it right then, but I would later that evening when I got home. "But what if you die before you get home?" he asked. I put him on my shoulders. He's a smart negotiator, and I'm a sucker.

Today, over our Sunday Chinese dinner (which I don't eat, of course), Zane asked me the dreaded question about what happens to people after they die.

What do I say? I don't want to patronize them and say we'll all go to heaven, since I remain agnostic about an afterlife. But I don't want to stress the possibility of a Yawning Void of Nothingness. That could devastate them. A friend of ours has a six-year-old son suffering through a premidlife crisis about his impending lack of existence, saying things like "I know God doesn't exist because He doesn't talk to me. So when I die, I'll be nothing. And I don't want to be nothing." Long crying jags follow.

I decided that admitting my ignorance was the best way to go.

"No one's sure what happens. Some people think it's like you go to sleep for a long time, but you don't dream."

They seem to be processing that one.

"And some people think we go somewhere called 'heaven,' which is a wonderful place."

"I hope that one is true," says Julie.

"And some people think we won't ever die."

Julie shoots me a look.

"There's a man named Aubrey de Grey, and he's got a looong beard." I draw my hand from my chin down to my stomach. "And he's a scientist. And he says that soon we will be able to keep our cells from getting old. Cells are tiny pieces of us and they build up garbage, and we just have to clean up the garbage. And maybe that would make us live forever."

"Like infinity years?" asks Jasper.

"Right," I say. "And there's another scientist named Ray Kurzweil who thinks we may be able to upload our brains into a computer and live forever that way."

"But we don't have to worry about any of this for a long time," says Julie.

Julie thinks I'm doing crazy talk. She tells me so later: "You're giving them false hope. You're feeding their delusions of immortality." Maybe she's right. But I've been steeping myself in books about the life extension movement. I've been reading about telomeres and sirtuins. I've read how some scientists think the humble lobster may hold some clues to immortality, since aging doesn't inflict damage on lobster cells. If not for outside forces like disease and predators, the average lobster might just keep on crawling along the bottom of the ocean for centuries.

The science of indefinite life extension isn't totally fringe anymore. It's not like Yeti or cold fusion. It's only partially fringe. So what's wrong with a little happily-ever-after, especially if it's got a little cutting-edge medical theory behind it?

Chapter 8

The Nervous System

The Quest to Hurt Less

I HURT MY SHOULDER the other day. I hurt it while lugging a sheet of drywall out of my apartment. At least that's what I tell people. Because I don't want to hear their sass when I tell them the truth. Which is that I hurt my shoulder kayaking. On Wii.

Yes, smirk if you must. Go ahead and marvel at my athletic ineptitude. It wasn't even a manly video game like Wii football or Wii rugby. It was recreational boating. But listen, I was paddling hard, trying to get a real calorie-burning workout, swerving around the yellow buoys, and, well, the damn Wii remote has no resistance. So I strained my shoulder. And let me add, I'm far from the only Wii victim. A simple Google search reveals dozens of articles on the problem, including one written by an orthopedic surgeon who recommends pre-Wii stretching.

And, in case it helps my cause, the shoulder is an easy part of

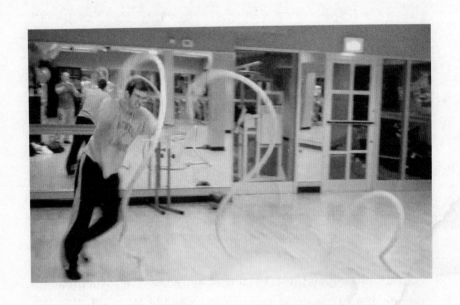

the human body to injure. It's a ball-and-socket joint, meaning it's got the widest range of motion, and the most chances for muscles, tendons, and ligaments to get tugged in the wrong way.

My shoulder injury has prompted me to devote this month to researching—and ridding myself of—pain. The first lesson: Thank God I was born in the age of painkillers. The majority of Americans are accustomed to living relatively pain-free lives most of the time. This situation hasn't been the case for most of human history. Pain has long been our constant, horrible companion.

Just contemplate the awful spectacle of surgery without anesthesia. Reading the absorbing book *The Pain Chronicles* by Melanie Thernstrom, you learn that doctors refused to tell their patients what day surgery was scheduled for. They simply showed up at the patient's house on a random Tuesday or Thursday for a surprise operation. Otherwise, the patients would commit suicide the night before. It was that bad.

Thernstrom quotes Fanny Burney, a British novelist who had a mastectomy in 1810 (performed, incidentally, by Napoleon's chief surgeon). Burney gave us the most vivid surviving description of predrug surgery. You might need anesthesia to read it:

> [It was] a terror that surpasses all description . . . when the dreadful steel was plunged into the breast—cutting through veins, arteries, flesh, nerves . . . I began a scream that lasted unintermittingly during the whole time of the incision, and I almost marvel that it rings not in my ears still! . . . When the wound was made and the instrument withdrawn, the pain seemed undiminished, for the air that suddenly rushed into those delicate parts felt like a mass of minute but sharp poniards . . . when again I felt the instrument, describing a curve, cutting against the grain, while the flesh resisted in a manner

so forcible as to oppose and tire the hand, then, indeed, I thought I must have expired.

Even after anesthesia was invented, it wasn't always used. Suffering, you see, was natural. When I wrote my book on the Bible, I read about the bizarre nineteenth-century controversy over women giving birth under anesthesia. Some felt it violated God's commandment "Women will give birth in pain."

Nowadays, pain has receded from our lives a bit. But we've got a long way to go. Chronic pain—meaning pain that lasts several months—afflicts 70 million Americans at a cost of $100 billion to the economy, according to a study by the National Institutes of Health Pain Research Consortium. We haven't yet found a suitable treatment for chronic pain. Pills work—but they tend to be addictive.

Reading about pain, I'm reminded, once again, that I want a refund on my body. Everybody should get one. Send this fleshy bag of bones and muscles back to the factory!

I'm not saying the body isn't amazing in many ways. It is. I could marvel for days at the design of the ear, and how it converts puffs of air into a Haydn concerto.

But at the same time, the body has many deeply embedded bugs. We're the result of ad hoc evolution and outdated hardware. And pain is one of the cruelest, most primal systems.

Pain is so unsubtle. Couldn't evolution have found a better way to alert us that we stubbed our toe? Rather than this sensation that makes us curse the day our mom and dad met at the college cafeteria? What about just having the toe throb gently? Or turn green? Or play a little ragtime number? I'd pay attention. I swear.

Pain is annoying and unnecessary, like getting an e-mail in all caps. It's like a six-year-old who alerts you every fifteen seconds that he wants Hungry Hungry Hippos for his birthday. Yes, I understand. Message received.

Maybe when we were slugs, we needed pain's brutish alarm system to pay attention. But now that we have cerebral cortices, pain should have been phased out.

Not to mention that pain is ridiculously unreliable. Thernstrom describes this problem with a wonderful metaphor. Think of pain as a guard in a watchtower. He rings the bell when he sees enemies. Problem is, the guard is "erratic, lazy, easily confused, fearful, a poor multitasker, and sometimes just deluded." Sometimes he'll ring the bell for no reason. Sometimes he keeps ringing the bell long after the enemies have been killed.

Pain can erupt with no cause, linger for years, even appear in a phantom limb. And here's one of pain's most sadistic qualities: If you suffer from chronic pain, it often doesn't ebb as the body heals. It gets worse. Pain begets pain. The neural pathways become smoother, the message stronger. It's a positive feedback loop that serves only to increase our misery.

Sharp Relief

My shoulder pain has gotten bad enough that I'll try anything to cure it. My general practitioner taught me some physical therapy exercises, which I do at home, using a pole as a very light barbell. No improvement so far. Julie gives me a massage every night as she reads her historical novels, which is somewhat helpful.

I've tried a makeshift Buddhist approach—instead of fleeing from the pain, I concentrate on it with a Zen, nonpartisan mindset. I say to myself, "Now *that's* an interesting sensation. The burning. The throbbing." I overthink the pain. But this strategy works better with short-term pain—a thumb jammed in a drawer, for instance—than it does with my lingering shoulder ache.

So today, I'm trying out new strategy: acupuncture. I find a place a block away—in New York, an acupuncturist is never more than a five-minute walk from your house.

And now I'm in the waiting room in the basement of a building. The door to the waiting room is propped open with a watermelon-size Buddha. I'm getting a whiff of that unmistakable Alterna Health scent. I can't pinpoint it—jasmine? frankincense? spilled kale juice?—but I always smell it at non-Western medical practices.

I fill out my forms and browse the pamphlets, which are clearly targeted at another gender. Example: a gluten-free tonic called Zenopause.

The acupuncturist calls me into her office. She introduces herself as Galina. She's a solid Russian woman in her sixties with bangs, a thick accent, and a white robe covered with words such as "Calm" and "Relax" in both English and Chinese.

"What brings you here?" she asks.

I explain the pain in my shoulder. She nods, jots down a note. Then she asks me questions for ten minutes straight, scribbling more notes.

"Do you sweat?"

"Yes."

"Which places?"

"Armpits and face."

I look around the office. It's dark, more like a Viennese café than an eye-squintingly fluorescent Western doctor's office. Asian fans and anatomy posters cover the walls.

After quizzing me on my sleep, bathroom, and eating habits, Galina gets up from her chair.

"You ready?"

"I'm ready. Except for the head. I don't want it on the head."

"Well, I'm doing the head."

Apparently, the customer-is-always-right philosophy wasn't taught in Galina's native Russia.

I groan. I have some long-standing neuroses about anything touching my head, much less piercing my skull. I'm irrationally afraid of brain damage. When I was a kid, it was even worse: The skull was off-limits. No friendly pats on the head. No soccer, with its insane practice of bonking the ball on your pate. And if Grandma came in for a kiss on the forehead, I would dart my head like Manny Pacquiao. Nowadays, I let Julie tousle my hair, but I'm still careful.

"The head actually has the least nerve endings," Galena assures me. "So it'll be the least painful."

I give a weak smile.

"One in a hundred people pass out. Maybe not even that. Usually it's the big guys." She laughs. She leads me to another chair in the center of the room.

"Which is more sensitive, one, two, three, or four?" She presses her fingers down hard on different areas near my bald spot.

"Three," I say.

"You know, acupuncture probably started in Russia," she says as she rubs alcohol-soaked cotton on my head. "The first corpse that had markings of acupuncture was found in Siberia. It was mummi-fied."

I'm not going to argue with a woman who is about to insert sharp objects into my exposed skull. She takes out a matchstick-size needle and pulls off its blue plastic cap. Then I feel a prick. Then a slide. There's a faint but distinct sound of the needle glid-ing through the various layers of skin. It's not too painful—about twice as bad as a mosquito bite—but the sound makes my stomach turn.

"You can look in the mirror if you want," she says.

I get up and walk carefully across the room. There it is, sticking out of my head like a tiny antenna.

As she presses on my skull again, Galena gives me a crash course in acupuncture theory. "It's about energy pathways. They are like roads in the body. And the energy can build up behind one part and cause the other parts not to have enough energy."

The acupuncture is like a tow truck that clears up the traffic jam. The chi (energy) can flow smoothly through the body's channels or meridians.

The channels are linked to different body parts. Today, she's working on the lung channel, which is linked to my sore shoulder.

Galena slides another needle into my head, and one into my left leg. She flicks the needle in my leg. It *boings* like a cartoon arrow going into a target.

After my acupuncture session, I head straight to the gym for a workout with Tony. "How many needles did she put in?" Tony asks.

"Three," I say.

"Three?" He laughs. "You got ripped off, my friend. On a per-needle basis, you got ripped off big-time."

Tony tells me his acupuncturist puts in forty needles, minimum. Even when he does acupuncture on dogs, which is his sideline business.

That's annoying. I didn't even get as many needles as your average Scottish terrier. Did Galena not think I was virile enough to take more than three needles? I could have at least hit double digits.

But here's the weird thing. Even though I was only poked three times, I notice something: My shoulder feels better. Not totally better. But a lot better.

For the first time in months, I can raise my arms in the air without a twinge. For the first time in months, I do shoulder presses with dumbbells bigger than hot dogs.

"This is amazing," I say. "The voodoo worked. It really worked."

So what happened?

To figure this out, here's a quick summary of the science's view of acupuncture.

Studies are split almost in half. Half show it works, and half show it doesn't. The studies show some cultural bias as well: Japanese studies generally come out more pro-acupuncture than American.

A couple of recent studies show that acupuncture works better than doing nothing. But so does "sham acupuncture," which consists of inserting needles in random places around the body.

So here are four possibilities of what happened today:

1. Chinese medicine is correct, and the needles restored my energy balance along my meridians. I'm too entrenched in Western thought to agree with number one.
2. The body does have pressure points that respond to needles, but science hasn't found the mechanism that makes them reduce pain.
3. Sticking needles into almost any part of the body (not including the eyes) relieves pain. Perhaps by causing a surge in opioids.
4. It's all a placebo effect.

My guess? And it's only a guess: a combination of three and four. And by number four, I don't mean to be dismissive.

Placebo Nation

The more I learn about placebos, the more I'm in awe. Humans are masters of self-delusion. It's one of our greatest gifts, right up there with speech and math and the ability to make soft-service ice cream.

Placebo—which comes from "I shall please" in Latin—is any fake treatment that gives patients real or imagined results. The placebo has probably been history's single most effective medical tool so far. It's cured more pain than aspirin, opium, and ice packs combined.

Placebos work on dozens of diseases and conditions. Pain, of course. But also coughs, epilepsy, irritable bowel syndrome, Parkinson's disease, and many others. They're effective about 30 percent of the time.

Though in the case of my children, the rate is much higher. It's amazing how a strip of sticky plastic will make my kids' pain vanish. Lucas will be howling about a stepped-on finger, but as soon as the Spongebob Band-Aid touches his pinkie, he's all smiles. My sons are so convinced of the magical healing powers of Band-Aids, they think they can solve almost any problem. A couple of years ago, when our Sony TV blew a fuse, Jasper stuck a Band-Aid on the screen hoping to revive it.

If you looked inside my sons' skulls, you'd see that the placebo makes deep changes to their brains, the same changes that would occur if they ingested real painkillers. Here's how Thernstrom describes it in *The Pain Chronicles*: "In a 2005 study led by Dr. Jon-Kar Zubieta at the University of Michigan Medical School, the brains of men were imaged after a stinging saltwater solution was injected into their jaws. The men were then each given a placebo and told that it would relieve their pain. The men immediately felt better, and the screen showed how: in the image, the parts of the brain that release their own opioid-like substances (endorphins, enkephalins, and dynorphins) lit up. In a sense, fake painkillers caused the brain to dispense real ones."

And it's not just pain neurochemicals. Placebos can cause other cellular changes. A study of asthma showed that a fake inhaler reduced inflammation in the lungs.

You could view placebos as depressing, I suppose. So much of medicine is a sham. Your brain is a three-card monte dealer playing cons on the rest of your body. But I don't see it that way. I find placebos uplifting and exhilarating. It means that taking action—no matter what that action is—might help you feel better. The key is just to get your aching butt off the couch.

I'm such a big placebo fan that I asked my general practitioner—a no-nonsense woman—to prescribe me some.

"Half the time I want real medicine, and half the time I want sugar pills," I told her. "Just don't tell me which is which."

"I can't do that," she said.

"Why not?"

"For ethical reasons," she said.

A shame. I blame the woman, who successfully sued her doctor in 1890 for injecting her with water instead of morphine, even though the placebo worked.

It should be noted that not all placebos are created equal. Studies show the mere shape and size of the dummy pill can make a difference in how people react. Capsules are more effective than tablets. Blue pills are better at mimicking soothing tranquilizers, apparently because blue is associated with nighttime. Pink pills are better fake stimulants. (Except among Italian men, where it's the opposite. The researchers' theory? Blue is the color of the Italian soccer team, and the color gets pill takers excited.) Syringes dull pain more than pills.

In short, the more elaborate the fake treatment, the better it works. Which is, I think, the secret to a lot of alternative medicine. Consider cupping. This is the practice of placing burning candles on the body, then covering the candles with cups. The lack of oxygen creates pressure that sucks the skin into the cups, causing flesh mounds to pop up all over your body. This supposedly draws out the toxins. With all that rigmarole, cupping has to do *something*, right?

The same logic could apply to acupuncture, explaining at least part of its efficacy. Turning yourself into a human pincushion is an extreme measure; the brain expects it to work.

Which brings up a question: Does the brain have to believe in the placebo for it to work? Do you need faith? Most studies have said yes. I still remember the sad day when I read that my favorite cold remedy, Airborne—those orange pills that dissolve in water— has little scientific data behind it. I believed in Airborne, and because of that, I'm convinced it stopped many runny noses. My faith evaporated after reading that wet blanket of an article. Airborne became useless.

On the other hand, one 2010 Harvard Medical School study purports to show that placebos work . . . *even when patients know they're fake*. Patients with irritable bowel syndrome improved when given pills they were told were dummies. Taking pills twice a day creates a "self-healing ritual," said the study's author.

I've experienced this so-called honest placebo effect as well. Though not with irritable bowel syndrome, thankfully. A few months ago, my glasses frames snapped during a wrestling match with my four-year-old. The lenses popped out. Lazy and stubborn, I wore the empty frames for a few days before getting them fixed. And here's the thing: I swear my vision was sharper when wearing my empty frames than without them.

If the "honest placebo" effect turns out to be true, I'm going to start a pharmaceutical company and market my new blockbuster drug, "Plazibo."

The Cursing Cure

Today, I ran across the park again to visit my grandfather. He was napping in his trusty recliner when I got there, and it took him a minute to emerge from the sleepy haze.

"What are you working on these days?" he asks.

I tell him about the health project, as I've told him a dozen times before. He nods his head. It's unclear if he remembers or not.

I tell him about my pain research.

"My favorite study shows you can alleviate pain by cursing," I say.

He laughs.

The study, which appeared in the journal *NeuroReport* showed that volunteers could hold their hands in freezing water forty seconds longer if they uttered expletives—it's possible the cursing activates the amygdala, a part of the brain associated with fight-or-flight response, which makes us less sensitive to pain.

My aunt Jane—who is visiting again from Maryland—says there's a lecture on the Internet about the psychology of cursing by Harvard professor Steven Pinker.

"Let's watch it," my grandfather says.

Jane finds it on YouTube, and presses play. Pinker starts with a quote from Bono—"This is really, really fucking brilliant"—which led to a Supreme Court case on obscenity. Pinker went on to utter the F-word with Mamet-esque frequency, as well as the C-word, the S-word, and every other offensive word you can think of, in noun, verb, adjectival, and adverbial form.

If ever I was going to listen to a string of swearwords sitting next to a ninety-four-year-old, I'm glad that ninety-four-year-old was my grandfather. Not that he swears a lot. It's just that he can take it. And, he is currently laughing so hard his eyes are watery.

He was—and still is—young at mind. He watches *Colbert* and *South Park*. He's fascinated by new things. He was an early adapter before there was such a phrase. I remember when he bought a video camera when they were shoulder mounted behemoths that looked like they could launch missiles. He loves the computer, the Internet, and cell phones.

And his friends? They are all younger than he—partly by default, since there aren't a lot of ninety-four-year-olds around. But also by choice. He's always preferred young friends. I'm not sure he ever accepted being an old man. At his eighty-sixth birthday party, he switched the numbers on his cake so they read "68." "Much better," he said.

My grandmother was even more of an age denialist. She rarely associated with people from her own vintage. "All they ever talk about is where it hurts and what's wrong with their bodies." She preferred my generation. She came to my friend Douglas's thirtieth birthday at a club downtown, the only guest born before the Korean War, much less Vietnam. She said one of the highest compliments I ever paid her was to call her an honorary member of Generation X.

I can't cite a study, but I wonder if there's a correlation between age denialism and longevity.

Checkup: Month 8

Weight: 160

Miles walked on treadmill while writing: 302

Meals eaten in front of mirror this month: 18
Miles run per day: 2
Biggest health sin: 27 candy corns in a single sitting

It's a mixed month. Some good, some bad.

Dietwise, I discovered purees, which I love. Carrot purees, broccoli purees, squash purees. I steam the vegetables, toss them in the food processor, and there they are, my brightly colored pastes. I find this adult baby food comforting, which I don't want to over-analyze. I'd rather point out that there's strong evidence that purees help you lose weight. They take up a lot of room in your stomach, making you feel full on fewer calories.

But my mental state isn't so good. I'm mildly depressed, and I'm not sure why. Perhaps it's been the rash of health problems in my family. Julie's stepdad had to have leg surgery, and her dad is having trouble balancing after his stroke a couple of years ago.

Maybe my mood's cause is more superficial. Thanks to my bum shoulder and my inability to lift big weights, my chest muscles have shrunk again, so I still look like a recovering heroin addict.

I decide I need something to lift me from funk. Which why I chose to try out a fitness class called "intenSati."

I'd been hearing about this eccentrically capitalized class for months. Friends of friends would not so much recommend inten-Sati as command it. "You *have* to do intenSati."

So on a Tuesday, I convince Julie to join me. She's agreed to come on one health adventure per week. She reminds me I should choose carefully.

"This is going to be worth it," I tell her.

The class is held at Equinox—a fancy gym where an attractive spokesmodel is giving out free samples of a new blueberry-flavored energy drink.

The hundred or so students gather in the heavily mirrored aerobics room. We grab our mats, and wait for our leader, Patricia Moreno. Patricia is the inventor of intenSati, and one of the most cultishly adored trainers in New York.

She appears. She's a beautiful, caramel-skinned woman wearing a head mike, a pink stretch to top, and carrying a notepad. She's also seven months pregnant, a fact that won't stop her from deep squats or high kicks.

She flicks the lights to red, giving the room a soothing feel, or a developing-old-photographs feel, depending on your point of view.

"We're going to have a great new program today!" says Patricia.

Whoops and applause from the crowd.

Patricia glances down at her notepad. She gives a five-minute speech about how you have to sacrifice to achieve your goals.

I glance over at Julie. Her arms are crossed. Bad sign. Julie doesn't come to the gym for sermons. She just wants to expend energy and fatigue her muscles.

And we do. After the speech, we give every part of our bodies a workout—and that includes the vocal-cords.

IntenSati, it turns out, isn't just aerobics. It's aerobics mixed with a Tony Robbins workshop and a Pentecostal service. It's fifty minutes of thrusting, pumping, jumping—all overlaid with shouted affirmations.

"I am never giving up!" yells Patricia as she squats and jumps.

"I AM NEVER GIVING UP!" we yell back, squatting and jumping.

"Are you in it to win it?!"

"I AM IN IT TO WIN IT!" We bend down, touch the floor, punch the air in front of us.

"I want it, I want it, I really really want it!" shouts Patricia.

"I WANT IT, I WANT IT, I REALLY REALLY WANT IT!" we holler back as we step to the side and kick.

The crowd—mostly women, mostly well toned, mostly glistening by now—are really into it, shouting loudly enough to raise the veins in their necks. I look at Julie. She's saying the words with all the enthusiasm of a third grader reciting the Pledge of Allegiance.

"Warrior pose!" shouts Patricia.

We jump and spread our legs out like a ninja.

"Every day, in every way, I co-create my reality!" she shouts.

"EVERY DAY, IN EVERY WAY, I CO-CREATE MY REAL-ITY!" we shout.

I'm trying to balance Julie's lack of intenSati spirit with my own zealousness, which is part earnest, part manufactured. I'm doing this somewhat out of guilt. I made Julie come, and I want to convince her—and myself—that it's a worthwhile hour.

I have nothing against affirmations, even overly complicated ones. Co-creating my reality? I can go with that. We do see the world the way we want to.

It's not a bad catchphrase. And I've been on the hunt for some good inspirational slogans ever since I had to stop using Nike's beautifully succinct "Just do it!" (I discovered that the advertising copywriter got the idea for the phrase from the last words of executed murderer Gary Gilmore. So I can't say it without thinking of a firing squad.)

Anyway, I'm committing myself to these affirmations. And I swear, over the course of forty minutes, I start to get more confident. My posture improves. My endorphins flow.

Yell this stuff in a room for long enough, and you start to believe it. I *can* do anything! I can write an epic poem! I can design a hydrogen fuel cell! Unfortunately, one thing I cannot do is convince Julie the class was worth her time.

"I feel like I was just at a Hare Krishna meeting," she says as we're packing up to leave.

Julie won't be coming back. Though for the next two weeks, she did incorporate intenSati into our lives.

"Can you hand me the business section?" she said the next morning. "I want it. I want it. I really, really want it!"

In the end, I probably won't be a regular intenSati-goer either. But I see its charms. Some level of delusional optimism is healthy. As long as that delusional optimism is balanced with a sensible understanding that we have pathetically little control over our fates. It's a tricky mix, but a crucial one.

You need both. Without *some* delusional optimism, you'll suffer from Depressive Realism. This psychological theory holds that the people with the most accurate view of the world aren't happier—they're clinically depressed. Studies show they have a correct perception of how much they control the outcome of events—namely, very little—and it crushes them. (Not all scientists buy this theory, but the ones who don't are probably, you know, deluded.)

If your worldview is too real, you might spend all your time in bed eating Bugles corn chips feeling overwhelmed and listless. You'll be too aware of all the thousands of factors toying with your destiny—from the weather to your genes to a misplaced pair of socks.

On the other hand, if you're too delusionally optimistic, you'll be unbearable. You'll refuse to save money or make backup plans. You'll invade foreign countries and expect to be greeted as liberators. Like everything else in health, you need balance.

Chapter 9

The Lower Intestine:

The Quest to Go to the Bathroom Properly

I'VE STUMBLED ACROSS some strange information in my health research. There's Capgras syndrome, in which a person believes that his mother (or sister or best friend) has been replaced by an identical-looking impostor. There's a disease called "pica," where the sufferer has an overwhelming desire to eat dirt, paper, glue, or clay.

But right now I'm being told the oddest, most baffling detail I've heard all year.

I'm in the office of Dr. Lester Gottesman in midtown Manhattan. And he's describing to me an elective surgery that he's performed not once, but several times.

It's for people who want to change the way they sound.

When they fart.

Yes, these patients want to change the timbre of their flatus,

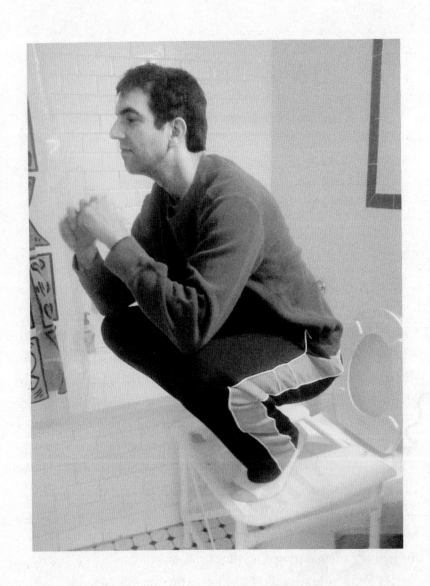

usually from a high pitch to a lower pitch. From a piccolo to a bassoon. Apparently, that's more aesthetically pleasing.

So he's done several procedures to tweak New Yorkers' sphincters. "I try to talk people out of [the surgery], but some people have a whole psychodrama about farts."

I'm not sure how to react to this information. Mostly, I'm thinking that if the revolution comes, this fact alone will make it hard to fault the insurrection. "Well, I don't approve of mass executions of the ruling class," we'll have to admit. "But on the other hand, there's that trend of plastic surgery to upgrade our farts. We really were asking for it."

As a committed experiential journalist, I also wondered if I should submit to the operation and become a baritone myself. But Dr. Gottesman says it has no known health benefits. Which is a relief.

But I do need to address other aspects of my colorectal health. I can't ignore my bottom. I've spent months obsessing about what to eat, but not a minute on how to take out the body's trash. It seems imbalanced. It seems unhealthy.

I'm not a big scatology fan, unlike my sons, who can amuse themselves for an entire afternoon by repeating the phrase "crocodile fart." So I'll spare you from an overabundance of detail in this chapter. This chapter will be somewhat soft focus, like the TV camera in a Barbra Streisand interview.

I found Dr. Gottesman because he's been included on *New York* magazine's Best Doctors list for the last eight years and has written, in his words, a "shitload" of academic articles.

When I first arrived, I filled out my paperwork in the waiting room, which had a sign that said NO EATING. That seems unnecessary. You'd hope that the word "colorectal" would dampen one's hunger for a chalupa.

Soon after, Dr. Gottesman calls me into the exam room. He's soft-spoken, so much so that I find myself leaning forward to hear him. He's got orangish hair, which is tousled in a just-woke-up way.

"Kneel there, pull down your pants, and lie on your stomach," he says.

I follow orders.

"Can you give me an estimate on the pain?" I ask over my shoulder.

"It shouldn't hurt too much. Unless you want it to."

I phone in a half snort, half laugh. I'm guessing proctologists have to memorize ten such responses for their board certification. Just as the Talmud must require mohels to make circumcision jokes.

After the exam—which hurt much more than I "wanted"—we went to his office for a debriefing.

I sat down across from his desk. He had on a concerned face.

"Do you read while going to the bathroom?

"Sure," I say. "Who doesn't?"

"I could tell you did. You have significant hemorrhoids. They're not huge, but they're not small."

This diagnosis seems spectacularly unfair. One of the least welcome pieces of news in my project so far. They can take away my Doritos. They can forbid me Diet Cokes. But reading on the toilet? That's practically in the Bill of Rights.

Dr. Gottesman is stern.

"Don't read novels on the toilet," he says. "Don't write novels on the toilet. If you keep doing it, then you'll have to get surgery. And hemorrhoid surgery is not fun."

Reading distracts you, causing you to sit on the toilet longer. Sitting on the toilet causes swelling of the veins in the anal canal. And that swelling results in enlarged hemorrhoids—a condition that affects more than 70 percent of Americans at one time or another.

I promise to keep magazines out of the bathroom. I then ask Dr. Gottesman some other common colorectal questions.

How often should I be moving my bowels?

Some zealous say we should go frequently and in great quantity. On *Dr. Oz*, I watched a gastroenterologist rave about sub-Saharan people whose three-times-a-day movements are "the size of my head." Also, Dr. Oz famously recommends that the poop be in the shape of an S-curve.

Dr. Gottesman—echoing the recommendations from the Mayo Clinic—is less specific. Anything from once every three days to three times a day is acceptable, he says. And the S-curve is fine, but not necessary.

How much fiber should I be getting?

A huge amount. The Institute of Medicine says thirty grams a day. Which is a challenge. An apple—one of the most high-fiber foods—has only three grams of fiber.

When should I get a colonoscopy to screen for colon cancer?

Unless I have a family history or symptoms (thank God, I don't), most experts recommend fifty.

Should I wipe while standing or sitting?

Sitting. It's easier to get fully clean, he says.

Should I get a colonic?

"They don't help, but they probably won't hurt." Colonics are supposed to wash away toxins that build up in your bowels. There's scant scientific evidence to support any health benefits. (Incidentally, as part of my project, I did get a colonic, but I've decided not to write about it at length. I didn't find it helpful or enlightening. I can tell you what it felt like, though: It felt like someone shooting water up your butt.)

Operation Squat

Dr. Gottesman's no-reading-on-the-toilet commandment is a good, if unwelcome, piece of advice. But the more I learn, the more I realize, it's only a half measure.

To have the ultimately healthy bathroom experience, I shouldn't be sitting at all. I should be squatting.

I first heard about the joys of squatting from Vlad, the raw-meat-loving caveman who told me I had a flat chest. He informed me that he goes to the bathroom by perching on the seat of the toilet. But since I'm a novice, I should buy an apparatus on the Internet to help position myself.

I dismissed his squatting lecture as caveman crazy talk. But oddly enough, there's bonafide evidence that squatting is better for you. I e-mailed Gottesman, and he backed it up.

As Daniel Lametti points out in a definitive *Slate* magazine article on the topic, the sit-down toilet is a recent invention, dating back to the sixteenth century. Lametti quotes a proctologist in *Time* magazine who said, "We were not meant to sit on toilets, we were meant to squat in the field."

Sitting puts more strain on the bowels than squatting, leading to an increase in hemorrhoids. Several studies address the issue. One Israeli scientist compared subjects who squatted over a plastic container and those who defecated on a high toilet. The squatters averaged 51 seconds per movement. The sitters, 130 seconds. And the squatters also rated the experience easier.

The most fervent pro-squatters say the posture also prevents cancer and Crohn's disease, though these claims remain unproven.

Following Vlad's orders, I found a squat-aiding apparatus on the Internet. It's called "Nature's Platform." Apparently, demand is high. The website was out of stock.

Regardless of the warning, I ordered it, and Nature's Platform arrived a few days later. The platform consists of a folding metal frame topped by a white plastic board with a volleyball-size hole in it. You assemble Nature's Platform yourself, put it over the toilet, climb on top, and squat, essentially turning your flush American Standard into a third-world hole in the ground.

I install my Platform before Julie comes home from a meeting. She heads to the bathroom. I wait.

"Not funny!" she shouts from inside. "Not funny at all."

She says that, but in truth, she's laughing. It's hard to resist the charms of Nature's Platform.

Julie gives Nature's Platform a test-drive while peeing, and pronounces it "interesting."

"Flowers are a more traditional gift," she tells me, when she gets out.

I've been using Nature's Platform for a couple of weeks. It definitely speeds things up. Though it does turn reading on the into toilet a dangerous acrobatic balancing act. Books are out of the question. Which would make Dr. Gottesman even happier.

By the way, after going, one other health tip: I make sure to shut the lid before flushing. Otherwise, an explosion of tiny droplets of bacteria-ridden toilet water will coat your bathroom walls and toothbrushes. You're welcome!

Checkup: Month 9

Weight: 158

Total steps this month: 230,000

Push-ups till collapse: 58

Days in which ate cayenne pepper powder in morning
   because a study showed spicy food lowers hunger: 12

Overall health: I'm finding the project exhausting—but oddly, mentally as much as physically. Dozens of times a day, I try to figure out what's the healthiest course of action. But often, I feel lost in the fog of conflicting advice.

Take the treadmill. After about three hours, my treadmill starts to stink like burned rubber. My son Jasper holds his nose when he's nearby. So are the positive benefits outweighed by these noxious fumes?

If I have an extra hour in my day, should I go to the gym or visit my family? All the health books emphasize the importance of family and friends.

Should I get a carpet because it blocks noise, or will that send allergens into the air?

When I have water at a restaurant, should I ask for a twist of lemon, because lemon juice lowers the glycemic index? Or demand that no lemon get within a yard of the glass, because microbe experts say restaurant lemon wedges teem with germs?

I bought a steamer, because you can't get much healthier than steamed vegetables. But my steamer is made of plastic. Am I making myself some hormone-disrupting broccoli?

I need to relax.

Chapter 10

The Adrenal Gland

The Quest to Stress Less

IT OCCURS TO ME THAT writing a book about health is not healthy. In fact, writing *any* book is bad for you.

There's the sedentary lifestyle (which I've curbed somewhat with my treadmill desk). There's the isolation—being alone breeds depression, which helps explain the absurd number of authors who've come to unhappy endings (Hemingway, Woolf, Plath—I could fill up the rest of the page).

And then there's the pressure. I'm way behind schedule. My publisher keeps reminding me of my deadline, and I keep replying that deadlines are *incompatible* with health. As are book releases. If and when my book comes out, what if I get the flu or an eye infection or something? I worry about that a lot. "You see the world's healthiest man?" they'll say. "He's the one in the corner with a hacking cough."

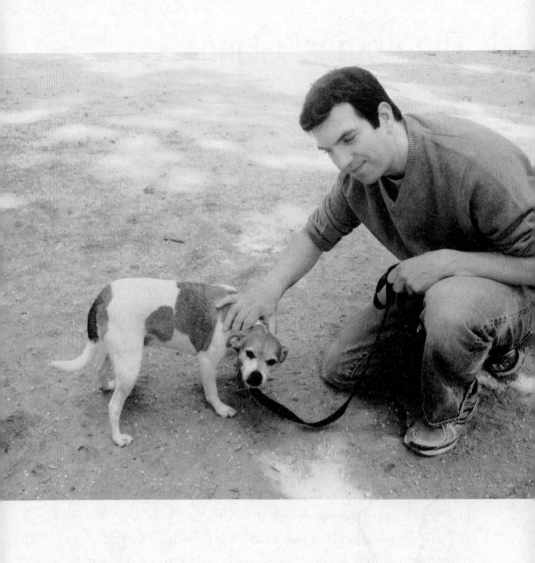

To combat this conundrum, I'm wrestling with stress this month.

Before this year, I was a bit of a skeptic. I was still too much of a Cartesian dualist to believe that stress was all that bad for your body. No more. Stress is not like vibes or auras. There's an Everest of data showing that stress wreaks all sorts of physiological havoc.

The term "stress," as psychologist Dr. Esther Sternberg writes in her book *Healing Spaces,* was coined by a Hungarian endocrinologist named Hans Selye. So obsessed was he with the concept, he had the chemical structure of the stress hormone cortisol carved into the stone above his front door.

Like so much else in the body, stress started out as a helpful ally back in Paleo times. Stress increases the heart rate, which is useful in the short term for running and fighting. It even helps ward off some disease in the short term. A 2002 National Institutes of Health study measured immune cell levels in skydivers just as they were about to jump. They had 40 percent higher disease-fighting natural killer cells.

But over the long haul, the high heart rate and constricted blood vessels suppress the immune system. The more worry, the more sickness. In one of many such studies, a researcher found that mouth wounds took 40 percent longer to heal when students were in the middle of exam week.

There's a big problem with acknowledging that the mind plays a part in physical disease. We're tempted to blame the patient. *Stop being so grumpy and you'll get better. You can will (or pray or think) yourself out of sickness! Buck up!*

This danger fed my skepticism about the bodily effects of stress and moods. It smacks of *The Secret,* that bestselling but bunkum-filled book that says you can wish those cancer cells right out of your body. The last thing a melanoma patient needs to hear is that they should "turn that frown upside down" if they want to get better.

Robert Sapolsky—author of the great book on stress *Why Zebras Don't Get Ulcers*—calls it a "lapsarian" view, "characterizing illness as the punishment meted out by God for sin."

And indeed, so far, science shows no link between cancer and stress. That's important to state, because much of America believes otherwise. Sapolsky cites a 2001 study where the majority of patients believed their breast cancer was caused not by genetics, diet, or environment, but by stress.

But when it comes to other health problems, stress gets trickier. Studies show a huge link between stress and heart disease. And studies also show that we can, to some extent, control our stress level.

At least for me, this leads to a horrible positive feedback loop of worry. If I worry too much, I'll increase my likelihood of heart disease. So I worry about worrying too much. And that increases my worry. Which makes me worry I'm even more at risk for heart disease. I need help.

Ho, Ho, Ho, Ha, Ha, Ha

It's Monday night, and I've chosen to go to a laughter club. I read about laughter clubs in *Time* magazine, and they seem like a relatively painless, if dorky, way to cut down on stress.

The club I choose is called "laughter yoga," led by a chiropractor named Alex Eingorn in his midtown office. Eingorn writes on the website: "It's free, but I'll accept $2 million donations with no questions asked."

Eingorn, it turns out, looks a bit like Mikhail Baryshnikov. He speaks with a slight Russian accent and is happy and welcoming, as you'd hope a laughter club leader would be. He wears casual blue Nike shorts and a sweatshirt.

There are fifteen of us tonight, ranging in age from early twenties to eighties, and we stand in a circle.

"Are you ready?" asks Alex. "Okay, drop and give me twenty."

We all chuckle.

"Any newcomers?" Alex asks.

I raise my hand.

"How'd you hear about us?"

"The Internet," I say.

A wave of laughs and titters. I like this room. This isn't what you'd call a tough room. This room could, in fact, be the easiest in New York City. I'm not sure why "Internet" got such a big reaction. It's association with porn? With geeks? Who cares? I'm just happy "the Internet" was considered an Algonquin-worthy quip.

Eingorn asks us to go around the room and say our names and occupations. And, he adds, somewhat unnecessarily, we should respond to each other with laughter. That will break the tension.

First guy: "I'm Tom. I'm an accountant."

There's some laughter.

Second guy: "I'm Steve. I'm a consultant."

More laughs.

Third guy: "I'm also Steve."

Big laughs. A callback.

There was a psychoanalyst (good reaction), plumber (huge one), and then me.

"I'm A.J. and I'm a writer," I said.

Everyone busts out at that one, rivaling the response for the plumber. This time I have mixed feelings. What's so funny about a writer? Is it really as funny as the plumber, an occupation known for clogged toilets and low-riding pants? Intellectually, I know the group is just following orders, but a deeply buried part of me feels as though they are mocking me. A writer? In this day and age? Time to dust off the résumé, pal.

For the newbies, Eingorn gives a quick intro to laughter clubs. The movement was started by an Indian physician named Madan Kataria in the mid-1990s. It soon spread all over the world, with a reported six thousand clubs in sixty countries. (A poster in the corner shows a record-breaking ten thousand people in Copenhagen laughing in a plaza on World Laughter Day, the first Sunday in May.)

We don't tell jokes, says Eingorn, because humor is subjective. We just laugh.

"We like to say, 'Fake it till you make it.' Force yourself to laugh in the beginning, and you'll eventually start laughing in earnest."

The health benefits are huge, he says. Laughter lowers the level of the stress hormone cortisol by 26 percent. A study said laughter therapy helped people with heart attacks improve 40 percent faster. And it's even good exercise. Laughing burns as many calories per hour as rowing.

I didn't want to bring it up, but Eingorn was slightly overstating the case. Studies have shown that laughter does indeed lower stress levels. But what about fake laughter? No one has any rigorous studies on that.

Enough warm-up. Time for the laughter yoga. There isn't so much yoga, actually. Just a handful of stretches.

Instead, the experience is like a cocktail party, where you mill around the room, exchanging witty repartee with the other guests. The only difference is that there are no cocktails and no witty repartee. Just the laughter.

And to keep it interesting, you laugh in different ways. We go through about ten different laughs over the course of the hour. In no particular order, there was:

- the "oops, I dropped a vase" laughter. Here, we mime fumbling a vase, then shrug our shoulders and laugh.
- the "I'm late" laugh. We point to our invisible watches and shrug our shoulders and give a carefree laugh.
- the explosive laughter.
- the snort-filled laughter.
- the "no-no-no" laugh. In this one, we wag a finger and remonstrate with our fellow laugher for an imaginary transgression.
- the laugh of retribution. "Sometimes in life you feel like a heroic statue. And sometimes you feel like a pigeon who is looking for statues to take a dump on. So we're going to be the pigeon." Here, we flap our arms, say "bok, bok, bok," momentarily squat down, then laugh.

I am faking it, not making it. I force myself to emit laughing sounds so I won't look like a grump. But I am mostly experiencing a blend of emotions: fascination that this throaty exhalation of air has evolved into a signal for joy, mixed with embarrassment that I'm making such a spectacle of myself, even if others are making the same spectacle. And occasionally I feel jealous at other people's laughing skills. This one guy—the psychoanalyst with the ironed oxford shirt—has a wonderful basso profundo laugh. One of the Steves—the one in chinos—is a full-body shaker.

"Good laughing," everyone tells them.

Most people's laughs fade slowly at the end of each two-minute exercise, but the redhead with tights can turn it off suddenly, like someone had tripped over her power cord. Her discipline makes me nervous.

"Ho, ho, ho, ha, ha, ha!" we chant as we do at the end of every round.

During the next exercise, we laugh while miming pouring water into an empty cup. I am laughing face-to-face with a sixtyish woman in purple sweatpants, when she leans in and says, "You look more like you're yawning than laughing." At least I think that's what she said. There's a lot of background noise. But I think she is criticizing my laugh, which does not seem in keeping with the laughter club ethos.

I purse my lips, annoyed. I don't like her technique either, frankly. Way too shticky for me. Lots of eyebrow work and jazz hands.

"Ho, ho, ho, ha, ha, ha."

"Woody Allen said that 'I'm thankful for laughter, except when milk comes out of my nose,'" says Eingorn.

No one laughs, not even in this room. I feel bad for Eingorn, so I muster a cackle.

Eingorn reiterates the importance of positive emotions: "As Norman Cousins said, we all know that negative feelings make you sick. If you're depressed, you can have a heart attack. Or you can die of a broken heart." Alex mimes a heart coming out of his chest and splattering on the floor. We laugh.

And now the sumo laugh. We all put our hands on our thighs and stomp around the room, giggling. At this point, I have a thought. What if an actual four-hundred-pound sumo wrestler came into the room, diapered and oiled, and started tossing all of us against the walls? It's not a particularly funny thought in retrospect. It's a little violent, in fact. But at the time, it must have broken the tension for me. Because I chuckle for real.

A young adult novelist catches me chuckling, and she starts laughing. And I start laughing harder. And we look at each other. And then I am really laughing. A bladder-straining bout of laughter, the kind I'd get in high school assembly during, say, the singing of a

Thanksgiving song, and which I tried to contain by thinking of my grandparents' funerals and my own eventual death. But here I don't need to contain it.

Ho, ho, ho, ha, ha, ha!

Eingorn wraps the class up: "The goal of the laughter movement is world peace. I know it's corny. But we believe that if you're laughing you can't be angry. And if everyone laughed, they'd stop being so angry. So let's take a moment of silence to say a prayer or a meditation and just think about world peace." I close my eyes. Someone titters, which I figure is okay.

I walk home, flushed, a bit elated, like I just had two Amstel Lights, but also relieved not to have to laugh on command.

Julie arrives home the same time as me. She'd taken a friend to a play called *The Scottsboro Boys* for the friend's fortieth birthday.

"How was the show?" I ask.

"I really liked it," she says.

"Yeah, I heard it got good notices," I say.

Good notices? Who talks like that anymore? I sound like I'm in a Damon Runyon story. I wonder to myself where that phrase came from.

Julie, God bless her, isn't going to let this slide.

"Yes, it got good notices," she says, laughing. "The press agents were very happy."

Now I'm laughing, too. It's not an explosive laugh or a sumo laugh, but it's a good laugh. She doesn't let it drop, mentioning the Stork Club, Walter Winchell, and J. J. Hunsecker. Julie beats the joke right into the ground. For that, I love her. No one can make me laugh like Julie can, not even Eingorn.

Magical Thinking

There's a great quote I once read, but I can't figure out who said it, despite intensive Googling. It's from a celebrity who was asked as he got off a plane, "How was your flight?" To which he replied: "Terrible. I'm exhausted from keeping the damn plane in the air with my worrying."

That's how I feel a lot of the time. I'm a master of magical thinking.

My general feeling is: If I fret long and hard enough about X, then X will not occur. If I don't fret, if I go about happily reading my *SkyMall* and chuckling at the Nicolas Cage movie, I'll be punished for my insouciance. As will everyone on the flight. In this horrible perversion of the Puritan work ethic, it's my *duty* to fret.

To properly engage in magical thinking, I find you have to think of every possible ghastly scenario. That's the only way you outsmart fate.

This ritual can be a tremendously time-consuming. The other night, Julie went to a movie with her mom. Three hours later, she still wasn't home. Three hours and twenty minutes—nothing. I called her cell phone. No answer. I checked the movie time. Just an hour and twenty minutes.

I had my work cut out for me.

Maybe she was killed.

Maybe she had an ischemic stroke.

Maybe there was a bioterror attack at the theater.

You've got to be thorough and cover even the most unlikely of scenarios.

Maybe she met another guy. Probably an old boyfriend—she went on a lot of blind dates back in the day.

Choked on the Twizzlers.

Fell on the third rail on the C-line.

I searched the Internet for New York crime stories. Nothing about Julie or a nerve gas explosion at the Loews cineplex.

Finally, three hours and forty minutes later, I hear the latch on the door click. I'm flooded with relief. But also a sense of victory that I got her home safely. Thank God I outwitted fate yet again.

Turns out the movie's star—Juliette Lewis—showed up unexpectedly at the end of the movie to do a Q&A with the audience. Some kind of buzz-marketing campaign. That was the big delay.

I know my worries were illogical and unhealthy. Stinkin' thinking, as the professional say. But my brain adores anxiety and clings to it hard.

A couple of weeks ago, I got some help from a reader named Bella from Portland. She e-mailed me that she'd read an article I wrote in *Esquire* magazine about outsourcing my life. I'd hired a team of people in Bangalore, India, to answer my phones and return my e-mails.

She wrote: "I was wondering if I could outsource some of my worry to you. You see, I am a high school senior, and I am working on applying to college. I've been stressed about where I will or will not get in, and how much financial aid I will receive. I ask because you said it was very comforting to have someone to worry for you. I thought it might calm me down to have someone worry my worries. Now, I have no money to pay you for my worries, but maybe we could make an exchange. I could worry about something for you, and you could worry about college for me. I'm a very good worrier! Almost too good . . ."

She'd worry for me? That's a great idea. I e-mailed her that she had a deal.

The next day I worried for her about the admissions guy at Vassar, one of the schools to which she applied. What if he had a bad chicken salad sandwich before reading her application? What if he had a fight with his wife? These things are so arbitrary.

She e-mailed me that she was worrying about the looming deadline for my health book.

"Today I worried about the length of February, in terms of how many days you have. But then I remembered that March and January both have an extra day, which makes up for February's lack, so that calmed me down a bit."

It's an absurd exercise. But you know what? Also highly effective. Every time I'd start to stress out about my deadline, I'd remind myself that Bella was on the case. Bella agreed it was working for her, too.

It's got all the upsides of worry but without the soul-sucking emotional toll. I can't recommend the worry exchange enough. Julie asked if I was worried whether Bella was cheating and not worrying on my behalf. So I might have to get someone to worry about that.

The Hair of the Dog

There's a law in New York that adults are forbidden to enter a playground unless they're accompanied by a child. A grown man can't just walk in by himself and loiter around the monkey bars.

Fortunately for me, there's no such statute about dog parks. You don't need a dog to hang out at dog parks. So I've been lurking around this dog run every day. It's a couple of blocks from our apartment, is about half the size of a soccer field, and has at least several dogs chasing each other in circles, regardless of the weather. I'm hanging out there because petting dogs is healthy. Several studies show it lowers your blood pressure and stress levels.

I spot an elderly man, maybe in his midseventies, sitting on the bench, his Yankees cap tucked low, his caramel-colored Airedale terrier bouncing and sniffing at his feet. I approach.

"You mind if I pet him?" I ask.

The man shrugs.

"Who's a good boy?" I say, scratching the dog's head.

"His name's Logan," says the man.

"Hi, Logan!"

I smooth the fur on his back.

"You know, petting dogs is good for your heart," I say. "Lowers our blood pressure."

"Huh," says the man. "I've had him for three years, and last year I had open-heart surgery and they put in five stents."

"Oh. I'm sorry to hear that."

I'm not sure what else to say, so I keep patting Logan's back.

"So you're saying I didn't pet him enough?" he asks.

I look up. The man's not smiling.

"Well, imagine if you hadn't pet him at all. Maybe you would have had ten stents put in."

"Hmm. Maybe."

I couldn't tell if the man is playfully sparring or angry. Was he about to sic Logan on my throat? I felt it was time to move on.

The evidence is solid that pets are good for humans' health. A study by the Mayo Medical Center found that dog owners had significantly lower cholesterol. A study by the Minnesota Stroke Institute said that people who owned cats were 30 percent less likely to suffer a heart attack (though 40 percent more likely engage in scrapbooking).

There are a lot of possible reasons: Touching lowers stress by raising levels of oxytocin. You're more active if you have a pet, especially if you have to schlep outside every morning to walk the dog. You meet other pet owners, and form social ties, which are crucial to well-being. Plus there are the benefits of an emotional bond with the animal itself.

As with everything good, pet ownership has its downsides, of course. A 2009 paper published by the Centers for Disease Control warned that sleeping with pets can spread pneumonia, cat scratch fever, meningitis, chagas, and even the bubonic plague.

After the Logan fiasco, I tapered off my visits to the dog park. I can't always be leeching off other people. My family needs our own pet. The problem is, Julie has allergies, so cats and dogs aren't going to work.

Instead, we decide on a fur-free pet. I asked Jasper what he wanted: A chameleon, he said. He liked the whole idea of a pet that changed colors. It's sort of like a slow-moving TV screen, I figure.

We ended up getting a beginner, not-quite-technically-a-chameleon chameleon. It's called an anole lizard. It only has two colors in its palette: green and brown. Jasper named him Brownie, with Greenie as a seldom-used middle name.

Brownie doesn't have a huge personality. He eats crickets and takes naps. There's not going to be an Owen Wilson/Jennifer Aniston movie called *Brownie and Me*.

But I think it's worth it. I love the look on Jasper's face when Brownie scampers up his neck and into his hair. It's a wonderful mix of joy, tenderness, and disgust. The Germans probably have a name for it, but I don't know it.

A Relaxing Massage

I often find myself whistling the Monty Python song "Always Look on the Bright Side of Life."

It's the tune sung by Eric Idle at the end of *Life of Brian*. He's on a crucifix alongside twenty other accused criminals, and he warbles: "When you're chewing on life's gristle/Don't grumble, give a whistle . . . Always Look on the Bright Side of Life."

All the stress-busting books keep telling me essentially the same thing: Look on the bright side. "Reframe," that's the word they use. Yes, you're on the slow line at the grocery. But think of all the times you've been on the fast line and never noticed it.

Reframing has its limits, and being subjected to the death penalty is one of them. But still, when you're not being executed, it also has its uses.

I was in the airport going to Sioux Falls on a business trip. I walked through the metal detector with no beeps or flashing lights. But still, the beer-gutted, sideburned TSA guy said, "I need to check you."

Ugh.

"Can you put your arms out?"

Annoyed, I refused to look him in the face. I was not going to give him that pleasure. I stared over his shoulder and pursed my lips. He patted me on the shoulders. Then the sides of my body.

I was a supernova of negative energy. But for what? Halfway through my pat-down, it occurred me: I'm spending a lot of my brain's bandwidth being annoyed. Is it so bad to have this guy touch me? Is he hurting me? He's just doing his job. In fact, doesn't the research show that human touch is healthy? It lowers cholesterol.

What if I thought of this as a free massage? It's kind of relaxing when he's patting my shoulders.

Get the TSA officer some coconut massage oil and a citrus-scented candle, and I'd have to pay him a hundred dollars.

At the end, the guy gave me a friendly pat on the back. A signal that I'm good to go.

"Thanks," I said. My government-mandated shiatsu may not have lowered my blood pressure, but it probably didn't raise it either.

Memento Mori

The ultimate reframe, I suppose, is to remind yourself that you're going to die one day soon, so stop being a petty little bastard. Renaissance painters excelled at these memento mori, and planted little skulls in the corners of their portraits as symbols of our fleeting mortality.

I've been a fan of the memento mori concept for a long time. A couple of years ago, I decided to get a memento mori screen saver for my laptop. I downloaded an image of a white bony skull, the kind you see in a *Hamlet* production. Whenever I opened my computer, there it was, staring at me with its eye sockets. I found it jarring, a buzz kill. Why should imminent death be so gruesome? So I got a more chipper skull. I plucked an image off the Internet of a multicolored, sweetly smiling cartoonlike skull that was probably painted by a Bolinas resident.

The new skull has done a good job over the years of calming me. At least until recently. It now has started to backfire.

Take my latest inconsequential crisis. I did an *Esquire* interview with this beautiful Colombian actress named Sofia Vergara, who plays the heavily accented, stiletto-heeled young wife on *Modern Family*. We had coffee, we chatted pleasantly. That's not stressful part. During the interview, she went on a rant about how weird Hollywood women look after they've had too much plastic surgery. She called Madonna's cheekbones "crazy." It seemed funny, and in character, so I put it in the article.

When the article came out, the gossip blogs claimed she had declared a feud with Madonna. Madonna's fans flooded her with vitriolic e-mails. So what did she do? She tweeted that the reporter (me) made up the quote. Then I started getting calls from *Entertainment Tonight* about the feud and my part in it.

I was furious. "I can't believe she claims that I made it up!" I told Julie. "I have it on tape. Why would I make that up? Why would I want to?"

"Why do you care? It's ridiculous. It'll go away in a day."

"No. You don't understand. The Internet is forever. It'll never go away."

She besmirched my reputation, such as it is.

I went back to my office and looked at my smiling-skull painting. It relaxed me a little. But not totally. Because the Internet isn't the only thing that threatens to go on forever.

As I mentioned, I'm obsessed with these books on immortality. It's coming soon, possibly in our lifetime, say some scientists. The latest estimate, according to a *Time* magazine cover story, is 2045. Gene therapy will keep my precious telomeres long and sturdy. Sirtuin will keep my muscles fresh. And Sofia's accusation will follow me around for thousands of years, like an eternal National Sex Offenders Registry.

Mortality is scary, but there's a comforting element as well, since you know there's a limit. Immortality comes with its own set of complications.

Time Management

One of the most stressful parts of my life is the lack of time in my day. Staying healthy is pretty much a full-time job. Consider this partial list of what I have to do every day:

stretching (10 minutes)
meditating (10 minutes)
chewing (10 minutes)
saying the 80 percent mantra before meals (this is where you
    agree to eat only until you are four-fifths full) (1 minute)

humming (3 minutes)

brushing teeth (4 minutes)

flossing (2 minutes)

keeping a food diary (5 minutes)

putting on moisturizer and sunscreen (2 minutes)

aerobic exercise (45 minutes)

anaerobic exercise (20 minutes)

memorizing word of the day (1 minute)

napping (25 minutes)

reading before sleep (10 minutes)

doing neck exercises (physician and author Nancy
Snyderman says we should turn our head side to side five
times a day to prevent neck pain): (2 minutes)

airing out apartment (2 minutes)

wiping down germy surfaces such as remote control, cell
phone, etc. (5 minutes)

doing crossword puzzle and other brain exercises (20
minutes)

taking stairs instead of elevator (2 minutes)

walking instead of taking the bus or cab (20 minutes)

steaming vegetables (20 minutes)

grilling salmon (20 minutes)

making salad (20 minutes)

putting on/taking off earphones repeatedly (1 minute)

spending time on social interactions (1 hour)

scrubbing vegetables to get off chemical and bacterial residue
(3 minutes)

taking supplements, including omega-3 fish oil; vitamin B12;
and coenzyme Q10 (3 minutes)

paying respect to older self (1 minute)

petting dogs (5 minutes)

refilling water purifier (1 minute)

having sex (not every day, and amount of time spent is
    classified, per Julie)

checking pedometer (3 minutes)

writing list of things grateful for (3 minutes)

getting ultraviolet light treatment with Philips Golite Blu
    Sunlight Therapy to prevent seasonal affective disorder (15
    minutes)

drinking glass of wine (10 minutes)

I'm always looking for ways to shave time from my schedule. One of the greatest days of my life? The day I figured out how to make podcasts play at double speed on my iPhone. It works great with NPR. I also enjoy listening to a full-body relaxation course on double speed—"now-relax-your-toes-now-relax-your-calves," though perhaps it defeats the purpose.

My time deficiency is why I was excited to read about a newish fitness trend: the hyperefficient workout. Twenty minutes a week. Not twenty minutes a day. Twenty minutes a *week*.

Welcome news.

On a Tuesday, I take the bus down to another eccentrically capitalized place, InForm Fitness, home of the fastest workout in the land. I climb the stairs to the second floor of a building in midtown Manhattan, a space once occupied by a tuxedo shop. When I open the heavy wooden door, I find the quietest gym I've ever been to. No blaring Black Eyed Peas songs. No sweaty Lycra-clad runners pounding away on whirring treadmills. No clanging barbells. It's like working out at an ashram.

The floor is home to a collection of sleek, white weight machines. Three other clients are lifting. And I don't see a drop of sweat on anyone's face. One gray-haired businessman is doing shoulder presses in his oxford shirt, his tie slung over his shoulder. My kind of gym.

The owner is a man named Adam Zickerman, a broad-chested former medical equipment salesman with a master's degree in genetics.

Here's his theory in a nutshell: The key to being in shape is to exhaust your muscles. Push them to failure so they can rebuild. Cardio is one way to do that: You can exhaust your legs by running three miles. But that's inefficient, plus there are dangers (knee problems, for instance). The best way to exhaust a muscle? By lifting heavy weights superslowly for about two minutes at a time once a week. You'll stay in shape, get toned, and lose weight.

It's a startling notion. But one I don't want to dismiss it outright: There's at least fifty so-called slow fitness gyms in America, with the support of a handful of academics.

I meet Adam in his office, and we talk fitness under the watchful gaze of a framed photo of Albert Einstein. I love Adam, partly for his enthusiasm, and partly because he's prone to making sweeping statements, always good for a journalist.

"Aerobics is a creaking edifice," he declares.

To him, mainstream exercise theory is deluded. It's based on superstition, cobwebbed tradition, and pseudoscience. It's like creationism, but with lactic acid and electrolytes.

One of the major villains of our time, according to Adam, is Jane Fonda, but not for her support of North Vietnam. "When we look back, I believe we'll know Jane Fonda and her ilk as the people who destroyed America's knees." He laughs, knowing he sounds extreme.

But he continues: "Why would you spend six to twelve hours on cardio, when you can get the same exact thing in twenty minutes once a week?"

Cardio defenders are fitness Luddites. "It's like saying that the only way to type a letter is with a typewriter. You could argue, 'When I was in college, I used a typewriter and I got through fine.' Yeah, it got the job done. But why the F would you use it when you have a word processor?"

Adam started his gym in Long Island in 1997, and over the years, has gotten an avalanche of publicity. He wrote a *New York Times* bestseller called the *Power of 10*. He's been profiled in *GQ* and the *New York Times*, and featured on *48 Hours*. Tim Ferriss writes about the slow fitness movement in his bestseller *The 4-Hour Body*.

Talking to Adam, I can see why. You can't help but get swept up. He's got preacherlike charisma. He speaks of the "fetishization of the Krebs cycle" and how aerobics release dangerous free radicals. He stands behind his desk and thrusts his arms in the air to make a point.

After an hour, he stops. "I think I pontificated enough for now. We should work out."

Off we go to the workout room. I sit down at a leg extension weight machine. We won't have to do the three typical sets of fifteen lifts. We can do it all in one shot. I'll simply lift eighty pounds slowly till I can't stand it any longer.

"Ten seconds up, ten seconds down. And then repeat. Your goal is to reach muscle failure. You'll be out of this freakin' torturous machine in a minute and a half."

I push on the foot platform with my sneakers.

"A little slower," he says.

I slow down to octogenarian speed, the speed of Keanu Reeves doing kung fu in *The Matrix*.

"That's perfect."

I'm pushing hard. Without the momentum to help me, the

weights kill my legs. I glance at Adam. "Don't look at me for sympathy," he says. He adds, mockingly, "Mommy, it burns!"

But, Mommy, it does burn. It's like having the flu and an eight-martini hangover in my thighs. I grimace and keep pushing. My legs start to shake.

Finally, Adam counts down five-four-three-two-one . . . and I'm allowed to let the weights down.

"Thank you for that," he says. I had gone all the way to muscle failure. "Failure is success," he says.

I do five more grimace-inducing exercises—including shoulder, biceps, and chest—and say good-bye to Adam till next week.

When I get home, I boast to Julie that I just did all my exercises for the week. She should try it instead of sweating on the elliptical every day at the gym.

"You're saying that what I do is bad?"

"Well, it's probably inefficient. And hurting your joints."

I expected her to roll her eyes, and maybe agree to give InForm Fitness a shot. But Julie is angry. Attacking aerobics is sacrilege, like taking on her family or her beloved Philippa Gregory novels.

"You find one study that says aerobics is bad, and you latch onto that one!"

When Julie is mad, she stomps. When she leaves the room, I hear the glass table rattle.

I went to Adam's gym a few more times, but in the end, I decide Julie has a point. I have to continue cardio.

First, frankly, it'd be a little anticlimactic for my project to settle on once-a-week workout. It feels like cheating, like taking a train up Mount Everest. It reminds me of what Adam said when I told him he should be a consultant on *The Biggest Loser*. "It's not good for TV. Twenty minutes and it's over. Okay, see you next week." No drama. No sweat equity.

Second, the science behind slow fitness isn't solid enough, at least not yet. It may turn out to be true. It's not inconceivable. But it needs more study. I pray it pans out. I'm all in favor of shortcuts.

Stress-Free Friendship

"I'm taking Alison out to cheer her up," says Julie.

Alison is sweet. She's been one of my wife's best friends since second grade. They bonded over their mutual love of *Joseph and the Amazing Technicolor Dreamcoat*. Alison happens to be going through a tough stretch. Her partner died seven years ago, and she hasn't dated since. Then her cat died. Then her other cat died.

"We're having dinner at about six-thirty."

"That's nice," I say.

"Do you want to come?"

I pause. "It might not be the healthiest thing for me."

My dilemma: Hanging out with a close-knit group of friends is healthy. But what kind of friends? To be truly healthy, some research indicates you want fit and happy friends. Your social circle has enormous influence on your own behavior.

Obesity, for one, is socially contagious, argue some scientists. A 2007 study in the *New England Journal of Medicine* found that "a person's chances of becoming obese increased by 57% if he or she had a friend who becomes obese, 40% if they have a sibling who becomes obese, and 37% if a spouse becomes obese."

Surprisingly, they claim this correlation was true even if the friends or family members were hundreds of miles away. The same study suggested that losing weight is also socially contagious.

Not that Alison is overweight. She's svelte. But the same two researchers (Nicholas Christakis from Harvard, and James Fowler from the University of California–San Diego) posit that happiness is similarly contagious. Happiness, they say, spreads like a virus even among people not in direct contact.

A happy friend increases your chances of being happy by 15 percent.

A happy friend of a friend boosts your chances by 10 percent.

And a happy friend of a friend of a friend lifts your odds by 6 percent.

The study is controversial. But if you think there's a grain of truth to it, maybe you should not associate with anyone who is sad or pudgy. Maybe I should cut ties with my friend who hates his job. Or my other friend whose husband left her for a coworker. Or anyone with a BMI over thirty.

Maybe I should skip dinner with Alison. That'd make sense in a cold-blooded Spock-like world, right?

But it'll also make me feel like a bastard. And just as important, when I'm depressed and fat, as I'm sure I'll be sometime in the next decade, I'll need the support of my friends, all of them, no matter what their waist size or serotonin level.

I don't explain my thinking to Julie, who has lowered her gaze and is looking at me over the top of her glasses.

I just say: "Yeah, I'll come. Looking forward to it."

Checkup: Month 10

Weight: 157
Bottles of flaxseed oil consumed this month: 2
Trips to Whole Foods this month: 8

Pounds lifted on squat machine (15 reps): 300
Minutes of TV watched per day: 60
Minutes of TV watched per day while standing: 30

Project Health continues to startle me with unintended consequences. This month's surprise: I've actually begun watching professional sports.

The last time I paid much attention to team sports was when I was a kid—the year my dad took me to the legendary Game Six of the 1977 World Series. He made us leave in the seventh inning to beat the traffic. "But what if Reggie Jackson hits a third home run, Dad?" "Don't worry. He won't." On the upside, we did have the subway all to ourselves.

But now that I'm feeling more connected to those parts of me below the neck, I've rediscovered spectator sports. I want to see how Amar'e Stoudemire of the Knicks sprints and jumps. I want to study how Roger Federer snaps his wrist on the serve.

This renewed interest dovetails with my sons' innate obsession with watching men bounce and throw spheroid objects.

Jasper and I tuned in to the Jets in the play-offs recently. And when they scored, Jasper laughed like Ray Liotta in *Goodfellas*, and I laughed with him, and we stomped triumphantly around the living room, doing coyote howls. So this is what all the fuss is about, I remember thinking. I'd forgotten the joys of tribalism. I'd forgotten the deep irrational pleasure of belonging to an arbitrary group.

As with everything I do now, the question arises: Is it healthy?

Maybe not. A study of German soccer fans found that heart attacks in men more than tripled during the World Cup on days the German team played. The stress is too much.

But another study, published in the *Journal of Clinical Hypertension*, says that it might depend on which sport you watch. Football raises the blood pressure, but baseball lowers it. The latter's nineteenth-century pace puts us into near-coma states.

And there's one more health benefit: Watching sports may be good for your brain. In a 2008 study published in the *Proceedings of the National Academy of Sciences*, psychologist Sian Beilock says that spectators' spatial reasoning and language skills improve when they watch sports. Which brings me to . . .

Chapter 11

The Brain

The Quest to Be Smarter

THERE IS NO BETTER TIME in history to be an idiot than right now. Never before have so many people believed that if you work hard and apply the right techniques, you can upgrade your brain and become a nonidiot.

For decades, intelligence was thought to be fixed from birth, like eye color. You're born smart or born dumb. You can jam more facts into your brain, but your basic intelligence—your IQ, your reasoning skills—remains static. But now? As University of Michigan professor Richard Nisbett explains in his well-respected bestseller *Intelligence and How to Get It*, we're starting to discover how malleable the brain is. The scientific term is "neuroplasticity."

According to the metaphor du jour, the brain is like a muscle. You can build its strength. You can keep it from withering with age.

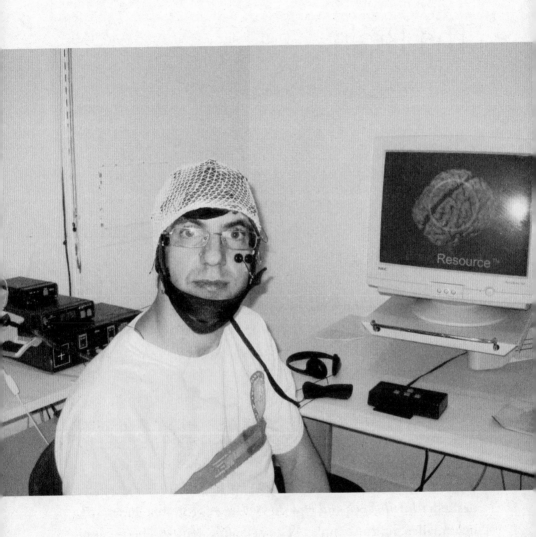

You can create new connections and carve new pathways among the brain's 100 billion neurons.

The key is to keep the brain active and challenged: do crossword puzzles, memorize poems, learn new languages. Meditation helps thickens the cerebral cortex. And make sure to eat the right brain food—namely, the good fats from nuts, olive oil, along with omega-3 fatty acids in fish. With these strategies, you can improve the brain in all areas—memory, creativity, attention, and reasoning.

It's a great and uplifting way to see the world. It's very American, too. Intelligence is not an aristocracy, with each of our brains assigned to be a prince or pauper from conception. It's a meritocracy. You work hard, and anyone can have a royal pair of frontal lobes.

But is neuroplasticity for real? Or is it just wishful thinking? The experts I talked to say it's a bit of both.

On the one hand, we're so enamored of the idea of self-improvement (me included, obviously), we latch onto promising studies and stretch them beyond recognition. Consider the so-called Mozart Effect.

Back in 1993, three University of California–Irvine professors did a study that showed that students performed moderately better on spatial reasoning tasks immediately after listening to Mozart's music. They were better at manipulating visual patterns in their mind. The effect lasted ten minutes. A short-term, moderate, and specific effect.

Before the study appeared, the Associated Press ran a story with the distorted thesis: Listening to Mozart makes you smarter. The media went nuts. Mozart CD sales exploded. Pregnant mothers pressed Mozart-playing boom boxes to their stomachs. And the taken-by-surprise scientists got death threats from rock fans.

Subsequent studies have either shown little effect, or else that

Mozart wasn't anything special. Any music temporarily improves spatial thinking. As the journal *Intelligence* put it recently, "Mozart Effect, Shmozart Effect."

And yet . . . if you cut through all the hype and *SkyMall* quackery, most scientists believe we can improve our own brains, at least somewhat.

And for my health project, improve it I must. The World Health Organization defines health as a state of emotional, mental, and physical well-being. I dealt with emotional last month. While I'm on this side of the Cartesian duality, I figure I should tackle the mental.

On the advice of brain experts, I'm following a list of mind-expanding activities.

- Do the crossword puzzle (several studies suggest that doing the crossword puzzle could help delay cognitive decline). I fill out the *New York Times* crossword puzzle on my computer every morning, or at least a few boxes. Crosswords have joined my list of Healthy Vices alongside chocolate and naps. Whenever I get a sidelong glance from Julie that says, "I thought you were so busy," I tell her, "It's for my brain!"

- Play logic games. I downloaded the allegedly scientific Brain Challenge onto my iPhone. You're given a Brain Trainer—a muscle-bound cartoon character in a white lab coat who berates you when you don't solve the logic problems quickly enough. "What's the matter with you today? You don't seem yourself." I deleted it. I don't need to be trash-talked by a bunch of pixels.

    I prefer the logic puzzles created by my son Lucas. They are a version of that game "Which one of these doesn't belong?" The trick is, instead of offering three or four items, Lucas only gives two options. He'll ask me, "Which one of these doesn't belong: the chair or the tomato?" "Chair?" I'll say. "No, tomato." It's more challenging than a Zen koan.

- Do the math. I tried one of the genre's most popular books, *Train Your Brain*, by Dr. Ryuta Kawashima. It involves a nightly routine of solving simple math equations. The promise is that the "delivery of oxygen, blood and various amino acids to the prefrontal cortex," will "result in more neurons and neural connections, which are characteristics of a healthy brain." The equations were so simple, even for a math idiot like me, I couldn't help but feel a sense of accomplishment, especially when my time dropped by fifteen seconds in six weeks. Plus, I like to exhale loudly while doing the exercises, as if I were doing some lat pull-downs. That makes me feel virile.

- Memorize poems. In his excellent book *The Brain That Changes Itself*, Norman Doidge argues that memorizing passages—as school children did in the nineteenth century had surprising benefits. "When students used to memorize poems, it helped them with the ability to speak fluently," Doidge tells me when I call him for guidance. I've been reading *Alice in Wonderland* to my son, so I spent a few days memorizing the poem "You Are Old Father William." I'm a sucker for any poem that rhymes "suet" with "do it."

- Become belligerent. Well, maybe that's not the way the researches put it. But that's what has resulted. One of my brain books says that one of the best ways to keep the brain sharp is to argue. Nowadays, I'm always looking for a fight.

Just today, I bickered with Julie about our Netflix queue, towel usage, and the placement of the apple juice in the refrigerator. I want it tucked out of sight so the kids won't see it, since it's so sugary.

Yesterday, Julie told me she read an article about how songbirds are being illegally hunted in Europe.

"Isn't that terrible?" she asked.

"Yes," I said. Then I saw an opening. "But let me ask you this. Is it any more terrible than people killing and eating turkeys or chickens?"

"So you're taking the side of songbird hunters now."

"No, I'm just asking, why should I have more empathy for songbirds? Because they look pretty and sound pretty? That's really unfair to ugly birds."

I then ranted about how we think it's okay to eat ugly animals: cows and turkeys. But if you're a beautiful creature, like a horse or a swan, you get a free pass. And we also treat ugly people horribly. Studies have shown that parents inflict less punishment on their attractive kids.

By this time, Julie had stopped listening, and I'm following her around the kitchen as she puts away glasses and bowls.

- Try new things. The theory here is that the brain is similar to a ski slope. The more times you perform an activity in the same way (shop at the grocery store starting at the left aisle, for example), the deeper the rut you make in your brain. The great, bumper-worthy phrase that describes it: "Neurons that fire together, wire together."

  If you want to keep your brain flexible and open to new ideas, you should eliminate rote, repetitive activities. A book called *Keep Your Brain Alive* has dozens of "neurobic exercises" to shake up your brain. I brushed my teeth with my left hand (wacky!). I took a different route home from the drugstore (superwacky!). I ate dessert first, then my entrée. (Get me to a psych ward!) I don't mean to be flip. There really is something wonderful about these exercises. They force mindfulness.

There's a tradition in Judaism that on the Sabbath, you should do things differently from the rest of the week. I once had an Orthodox Jew describe to me how she took this edict to mean that even lipstick should be applied in a new way—counterclockwise instead of clockwise. And this small tweak reminded her to focus on how pleasing the putting-on-lipstick ritual can be.

Of course, nonstop mindfulness is exhausting. You need a little dull repetition for balance. And there's another danger as well. When Julie found out that I had committed myself to embracing new things, she took full and cruel advantage. "We're going to try Momofuku," she said, referring to a trendy restaurant I've been avoiding. "I know it's loud, but you've never been there before. You should go. For your brain."

Testing My Brain

I decide to seek professional assistance. The Brain Resource Center in New York's Upper West Side promises to help my brain reach "peak performance."

On a Thursday morning, I meet with Dr. Kamran Fallahpour, a 48-year old neuroscientist with a trace of an accent from his native Iran.

Our first task, he says, will be to assess my brain. Kick its tires.

Minutes later, I'm sitting in a spare white room with a lot of stuff on my head. There are squirts of maple-syrupy hair gel. There's a rubbery contraption that resembles an Amelia Earhart aviator cap, with dozens of electrodes sticking out of it. All that is topped by a white hairnet.

The equipment is meant to track my brainwaves and eye movement as I go through three hours of mental games and quizzes. Dr. Fallahpour dims the lights; I slip on the headphones and focus on the computer screen.

My first task is to stare at a red dot for six minutes. I stare, and I stare. Dr. Fallahpour tells me I can't clench my jaw. It might throw off the reading. So my mouth is ajar. I look dumb. I feel dumb. Will this affect my score?

I do mazes, I memorize word lists, I arrange letters on a checkerboard pattern. I study photos of random faces and try to discern their emotions—even as a horrible gunshotlike noise blasts in my ear to distract me.

The test's narrator is a British man with a voice that's both reassuring and condescending.

"Well done," he says after each task, even if I flubbed it.

On another test, I have thirty seconds to say—out loud—all the words I can think of that start with the letter *F*. I begin with the perfectly acceptable "father, fancy, frankfurter." But inevitably, my brain starts working blue. Do I say the F-word? What about a particularly offensive slur for gay men? I was torn between my conscience and my competitive side. My competitive side won.

A week later, I return to Dr. Fallahpour's office to go over the results.

"Do you want the bad news first or the good news? I always tell people that the bad news is actually good news, because then we know how to treat it."

I'd rather have the regular old good news.

"Overall, you have no abnormality in the cognition areas."

He clicked on his Mac and pulled up my file. It showed charts with frenzied zigzag lines, and grape-size pictures of my brain glowing in red or yellow or green.

I did well on the verbal fluency, possibly because I resorted to slurs.

"You're in the right job," he says.

And the bad news?

"There's a little bit of slowing in the frontal sites. It could mean that you have some problems with executive function and parts of attention. Also in the affective area, you may have trouble with moods."

I'm also, I discover, terrible at memorizing word lists. Oh, and NASA should think twice before hiring me to help with liftoffs— I'm in the eleventh percentile for counting backward.

So . . . a mix.

"Overall, you have a pretty good brain," he says. Above average in many ways, below average in others.

My brain is not a Lamborghini. It's more like a Lexus, or a Toyota.

It's decent. I kind of expected that, but it's a little disappointing to hear it from a guy in a white lab coat. A little part of me still clung to the delusion that Dr. Fallahpour would burst through the door, clutching the results and saying, "I've never seen anything like this! Your brain is a national treasure!"

The Nerd-vs.-Jock Fallacy

I've always liked stories about eggheads versus jocks. When reading the Bible, I came to see David versus Goliath as a sort of prequel to *Revenge of the Nerds*. On one side, you had big dumb 'roided-out Goliath. And on the other side, skinny but smart David with a sling instead of a pocket protector. Everyone assumes David's going to get crushed. But clever David uses his high IQ to pummel the blockhead Goliath, and then goes off with the hot cheerleaders. Or at least he gets to marry eight wives, the biblical equivalent.

You can even view history as a nerd–jock battle for supremacy. In his book *American Nerd*, writer Benjamin Nugent argues that tensions rose when the industrial revolution forced men indoors and into unmanly, chair-bound jobs. Some men felt they had to reassert their virility.

So the split became more extreme: In one corner, you had folks like our jockiest president, outdoorsman Teddy Roosevelt, who railed against young men with shoulders "sloped like a champagne bottle." And in the other corner, you have people like geek hero Marcel Proust, a champagne-shouldered Frenchman who rarely left his bed during the decade he wrote his masterpiece.

As you can imagine, my friends and I always empathized more with the champagne-shouldered, bookish side. My motto: a sound mind in an unsound body.

But this project has been a shock to the nerd's-eye worldview. Because the stereotype of the smart nerd and the dumb jock is not accurate. Quite the opposite. Scientifically speaking, it's more accurate to talk about the smart jock. Aerobic activity increases brainpower. Which seems unfair. Nature doing another one of her cosmic jokes.

Fortunately for the skinny and uncoordinated, you don't need to be an all-star rugby player to boost your brainpower. Any movement, any type of exercise works. (The sales guy at my gym coaches a Quidditch team, a good option for the athletically inclined dweeb.)

The expert on exercise and intelligence is John Ratey, a Harvard professor and author of the book *Spark: The Revolutionary New Science of Exercise and the Brain*. Exercise, argues Ratey, improves your brain in both the short term (you're sharper for the couple of hours after aerobic activity) and the long-term (it staves off brain aging and Alzheimer's). It bucks up the brain in all sorts of areas, including focus, memory, mood, and impulse control.

There are dozens of studies on exercise, so I'll just pluck one out to give a taste. A study in the *Research Quarterly for Exercise and Sport* found that Georgia students who did forty minutes of daily exercise showed twice as much academic improvement as those who did twenty minutes a day. Those who got no exercise showed no improvement. Ratey lists dozens of similar studies in his book.

These findings make evolutionary sense. As Ratey says "While tracking their prey, our ancestors needed to have the patience, optimism, focus and motivation to keep at it. All these traits are influenced by serotonin, dopamine and norepinephrine." So we evolved to have higher levels of these chemicals when we walk or run.

On a cellular level, Ratey says, exercise increases neuroplasticity, blood flow, and levels of a protein called "brain-derived neurotrophic factor" (BDNF), which he nicknames "Miracle-Gro for the brain." If only Albert Einstein had an elliptical machine in his office, he might have cracked the Grand Unified Theory.

It would stand to reason, then, that those on sports teams would also be academic superstars. Except for one complicating factor: Jocks may not spend enough time studying. There are only so many hours in a day.

I haven't found any rigorous studies on school sports teams and GPA. But Ratey says kids on the lacrosse and soccer teams are generally above-average students, but those on football and basketball teams are not. They are too busy being "kings of the school." It's a theory I'm surprised hasn't gotten him beat up by high school football players.

Thanks to my treadmill desk, I'm sort of already combining thought and movement. (I'm up to mile 652, by the way.) But after reading Ratey's book, whenever I come to a hard problem, I do some jumping jacks to try to dislodge the solution from my brain. Sometimes it works, if only by waking me up.

A couple of weeks ago, I had to make a presentation in front of a bunch of intimidatingly smart people. I spent the ten minutes prespeech jogging in place backstage, though I stopped whenever anyone walked by.

Neurofeedback

I'm back at the Brain Resource Center for my cerebral workout. I sit in Dr. Fallahpour's black leather chaise longue, my eyes trained on a computer screen, five electrodes dotting my scalp. The screen has three vertical bars—blue, red, and green—that bounce up and down in response to my brains electrical activity. My job is to keep the bars inside their target zones.

How? It's hard to explain. "Think of it this way," says Fallahpour. "It's like one of those freeway signs that shows your speed in real time. It says you're going seventy-five mph in a fifty-mph zone, and you slow down."

If my brain nudges the bar above the line, I get a reward: relaxing Tibetan chimes through my headphones.

This regimen is neurofeedback, and Dr. Fallahpour is one of the country's experts on it. Neurofeedback, the idea that can learn to control your brainwaves to improve your concentration and lower your stress, is a controversial procedure. It's far from proven science, and some dismiss it as flaky. But there's some evidence that it might be useful, including a study by the National Institutes of Mental Health that found it could help combat attention deficit hyperactivity disorder in kids. A Stanford experiment has used neurofeedback involving brain imagery to alleviate some chronic pain.

It's a strange feeling to try to manipulate your brain waves. "Okay, now focus on the sounds of the bells," I say to myself. That seems to work. The bells chime, the bar stays up. So I tell myself, "Let's make a note of that strategy. Concentrate on the bells." But as soon as I take myself out of the moment and make a note of the strategy, the bells go silent and my bar drops. It's like meditation turned into a video game.

I did neurofeedback a half-dozen times, not as many as Fallahpour recommended. So many body parts, so little time. What I did, though, I liked. I always left feeling calm but energized, like I'd just had espresso but with no jitters.

Overall, after my month of neurofeedback and neurobics and math and arguments, do I feel like my brain is less flabby? It's hard to quantify, but . . . yes, a little. I'm faster at math problems. I took an online intelligence test and scored 23 percent better at the end of the month. I can memorize poems more quickly. I played the card game hearts last weekend. Usually, I'm happy to play on hunches and vague approximations. But this time, my well-toned brain felt up to counting cards. I still lost the game, but I felt more precise doing it.

It could all be the placebo effect. But as I've said before, the placebo effect is a godsend.

Memories of My Grandfather

I go to lunch at my grandfather's on a chilly Thursday. I open the door and spot him in his usual pose, sunken deep in his recliner, his slippers up, watching CNN. He smiles and gives me his signature raised-fist salute.

With his daughter Jane's help, my grandfather heaves himself up and shuffles over to the lunch table.

"We went out to dinner last night, didn't we, Poppy?" Jane says as we settle in.

"Where'd you go?" I ask my grandfather.

He pauses, searching his brain.

"Well, I know I had something to eat, so that's a start," he says, then chuckles.

My grandfather's memory is slipping away. But it's a selective vanishing—only for recent events. Any story that happened in the fifties and sixties—he knows it cold. This is officially called "Ribot's Law," named for the French psychologist who first studied it. The more times we recall a memory, the more encoded it becomes. Recent memories haven't had time to gel into the brain's circuitry.

And in my grandfather's case, Ribot's Law means that visitors spend a lot of time reminiscing about the distant past. Which is okay by me, even though I've heard the same stories a dozen times.

Today, we talk about the time my grandfather bought a pet alligator for my aunt Kate. They kept it in the bathtub until it nipped a guest and had to be given to the Bronx Zoo.

A mention of Egypt leads to his favorite Africa story. I know it so well, I could recite it in stereo with him. In 1959, my grandfather helped organize what's called the "Airlift to America." The goal was to get hundreds of Kenyan students to study in United States colleges and then have them return home to lead their country. My grandfather raised money in New York, then, on two days' notice, he flew to Kenya to conjure up some more.

He didn't even have time to get his shots, so he took a syringe and a bottle of refrigerated medicine with him on the plane. He later forgot the medicine in the Nairobi hotel fridge. "I think it's still there today," he says, every time he tells the story.

He bounced across unpaved roads in a Jeep to spread the word to Kenyan villages. He became the proud owner of a goat in a local auction—which he then donated to the cause.

My grandfather wrote back home that the experience was "as inspiring as anything I have ever seen. Words cannot do justice to the reverence these people showed for education."

My grandfather and his partners raised enough cash to charter two planes that carried eight hundred students from Nairobi to New York. One of those students lived at my grandparents' house in Riverdale for a year while he studied economics at Columbia.

More students longed to study in America than could fit on the planes. So the foundation provided scholarships to several other Kenyans. One of those students ended up at the University of Hawaii. His name was Barack Obama Sr.

My grandfather—a lifelong Democrat—still gets misty-eyed when Barack Obama Jr. gives a speech on TV. What a feeling that must be, to be so enmeshed in history. In 2009, an author named Tom Shachtman wrote a book called *Airlift to America*. My grandfather keeps it on the living room coffee table.

It might be pushing it, but I wonder if the Africa trip—and his other charity work—is one secret to my grandfather's longevity. Several studies argue that charity is good for your health. One MRI study showed that giving to charity lights up the pleasure centers of the brain. It's been called "helper's high." A 2004 Johns Hopkins study concluded that volunteering slows mental and physical aging.

You're more engaged, more challenged physically and cognitively.

After he finishes the Obama story, I check my cell-phone clock. I have to leave.

"Can you give me a ride?" asks my grandfather.

"Where are you going?" Jane asks him.

He pauses. "Where I was before."

"You've been here all day," she says. "This is your home."

"Oh," my grandfather says. "Right."

The mist seems to clear, at least momentarily, and he gives me another raised-fist salute.

Checkup: Month 11

I went to EHE for a checkup. I figure I'm about at the halfway point of Project Health—I always pictured it as a two-year venture (my body is a fixer-upper). Here are the results:

> My weight: 157 pounds, down from 171.8. Almost fifteen
> pounds. Not bad.
> Total cholesterol, dropped from 134 to 129.
> HDL (the so-called good cholesterol) spiked from 41 from 45.
> LDL (bad cholesterol) sank from 77 to 68.
> My iron-binding capacity is down to normal range.
> Blood pressure is down to 98/68 (it was previously at 110/70).
> My body fat percentage took a crazy tumble: down from 18.4
> percent to 8.0 percent. Nice.
> Pulse down from 64 to 55.

On the downside, I've got a mild hernia, and my doctor—a sweet-natured Indian woman—tells me that I shouldn't lift heavy weights. A serious problem since I'm trying to bulk up.

Overall, I'm getting healthier, which is good. I'm bucking the pull of gravity and entropy.

But I don't think I'm the healthiest person alive. Not yet. My body has lost some of its marshmallowness and gained some sharp lines, but it's still wiry. My pecs wouldn't measure up at your average beach, even those far from the Jersey Shore.

But more troubling, I have hundreds of things left on my fifty-three-page to-do list—which has now grown to seventy pages. I'm worried I'll never come close to finishing. Many body parts remain: my back, my feet, my skin.

Not to mention my surroundings. From what I've been reading, there's the distinct possibility that my apartment might be slowly killing me and my family. Marti's coming to town. Maybe she can detoxify our living quarters.

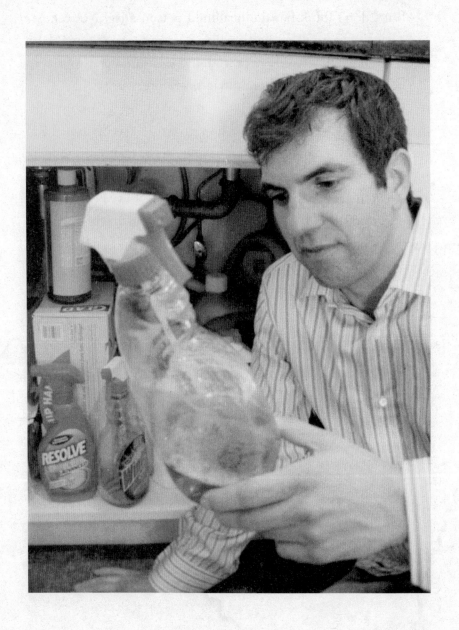

Chapter 12

The Endocrine System

The Quest for a Nontoxic Home

I HONESTLY DON'T KNOW WHAT to think about the toxins issue. One day I'll read books with horrifying titles like *Slow Death by Rubber Duck*, which argue that toys are made from endocrine-disrupting plastics that will cause my boys to grow breasts the size of Katy Perry's when they're twelve. These books warn my food will poison me, and my shampoo will give me scalp cancer.

The next day, I'll read that these fears are overblown, and the science has proved nothing of the sort. I need to figure out the truth.

To represent the anti–rubber duck side, I've called in my aunt Marti. Marti has a few opinions about health—and one of her main causes is toxic chemicals. I ask her to do a sweep of our apartment. She agrees.

Marti arrives on a Thursday morning wearing her trademark purple scarf and a backpack. She's in town to visit my grandfather.

"How was your flight?" I ask.

"Not bad, considering," she says.

Airplanes are always a challenge. She needs to carry her raw organic vegetables with her, but the TSA tried to confiscate the ice pack. She won't go near scanners, and she comes armed with a newspaper clipping to show the officers that they might cause cancer. Also, the flight attendant's cologne made her gag.

Marti acknowledges she's a character. She signs her e-mails "Your eccentric aunt Marti." But I don't want to dismiss her as a whack job. Well, sometimes she's a whack job, like when she went through a phase called "solar gazing," which is basically looking at the sun every day for thirty seconds to absorb some of its good energy. Staring at the sun. With your eyes.

But other times, she's years—and even decades—ahead of the curve. She warned us all about secondhand smoke when most dismissed it as alarmist babble. She's been promoting the health benefits of vegetarianism long before mainstream nutritionists started advocating a plant-based diet. Plus, she looks about twenty years younger than her sixty-two years. And she hasn't gotten sick in eight years.

Okay, let's go to work.

We start in the kitchen. Our sink has a bottle of strawberry-scented anti-bacterial soap.

"No, no, no," says Marti. "Anything that says 'antibacterial' is a poison. Just conceptualize skull and bones on it." Many believe triclosan in anti-bacterials is an endocrine disrupter and allergen. Marti says we need to buy organic vegetable-based soap.

We move on to the cleaning fluids under the sink. She picks up Mr. Clean Bath Cleaner and takes a sniff. She recoils like she's

smelled a rotting corpse. "Let me get out my oregano." She keeps
a vial of organic oregano oil in her backpack, which she dabs onto
her wrists to counteract the Mr. Clean nasal assault. I should be
cleaning with vinegar and organic baking soda.

And on it goes for another forty-five minutes.

My sunscreen and deodorant are tainted. They have parabens,
which cause endocrine disruptions and cancer.

My store-bought clothes have been treated with chemicals, and
need to be replaced with hemp, bamboo, or organic cotton fibers.

The plastic Keith Haring shower curtain with its abundance of
phthalates elicits a shriek. There might be a link to liver cancer and
lowered sperm production.

Having a microwave is like keeping a loaded gun under my
kids' pillow.

And my refrigerator is like a Superfund site. "Oh my God!
This is child abuse," she gasps, when she spots our chemical-laced
American Cheese.

She opens a drawer to find nonorganic cucumbers and blueberries. Pesticides used in nonorganic farming can cause everything
from cancer to ADHD.

"You don't have Wi-Fi, do you?"

I sheepishly acknowledge we do.

"That's like having a mini cell tower in your house!"

She says that a Canadian study showed that Wi-Fi distorted the
growth of Dutch ash trees. Marti thinks electromagnetic pollution
is an underappreciated health hazard. Wi-Fi is terrible, but even
old-fashioned wires emit harmful rays. In her own home, she hired
a worker to put all her wires—computer, phone, printer—behind a
wall.

We move onto the living room. She peeks under our Pottery
Barn lamp. As she expected, one of those fusilli-like CFL light

bulbs. "This gives off a small vapor of mercury. You need to take it to the toxic waste dump."

"I thought I was being environmentally responsible."

"You need to get an LED light bulb."

She points to a small arrangement of roses I'd gotten Julie for our anniversary.

"Those are toxic. Commercial flowers are sprayed with all kinds of chemicals."

"Doesn't the FDA protect us?" I ask.

"They're years behind. Remember when the government said tobacco was just fine for you? They said it soothed the nerves."

Julie comes into the kitchen to get some coffee.

"I just hope he doesn't have to get rid of me."

"Do you have metal fillings?" Marti asks Julie. "Because assuming you and A.J. are still intimate, you're sharing the toxins in your mouth."

Julie only has one filling, and it isn't metal.

"She's probably okay, then," Marti says to me, smiling.

I'm also lucky I don't have a car. The upholstery on car seats is on Marti's list of hazardous substances. Many have the flame retardant Deca, which has been linked to learning deficits. In fact, here's how committed Marti is to living a toxin-free life: When she bought her Toyota Corolla, she left the car on the street with the window open for *six months* before she drove it. Six months to let the upholstery emit its noxious gases.

After a raw food lunch, Marti goes to visit grandpa, and detoxify his house. I hug her good-bye, even though I probably transferred all sorts of chemicals onto her.

Better Living Through Chemistry

For equal time, I decide to have lunch with the anti-Marti. A couple of weeks ago, a mutual friend introduced me to a man named Todd Seavey. He works for a company called the American Council on Science and Health (a job he would later leave to work at Fox Business Network). The ACSH is a libertarian-leaning group that battles against what its members see as irrational fear of chemicals.

I'm already seated at an Italian restaurant when Todd arrives.

"How are you doing?" I ask as he pulls in his chair.

I was expecting some variation on "fine" or "pretty good." Instead, I got a three-minute mindspew about his horrible morning: A scientific journal has announced that it won't print studies funded by tobacco, which Seavey sees as a dangerous precedent, one that will grind science to a halt, not to mention that Big Pharma has been unfairly maligned even though they have been the main engine boosting life spans during the last fifty years. "I used to think Ayn Rand was describing a worst-case scenario. But it's coming true. They're regulating businesses out of existence." He lifts up his water glass. "Here's to the slow death of civilization."

I raise my glass tentatively, not sure what else to do.

Seavey—thin, dirty-blond hair, looks a bit like the actor Eric Stoltz—has worked for the Council on Science and Health for seven years. It's clearly a pro-industry group. But I don't want to caricature them as apologists for corporate America. For instance, they also take a strong antitobacco stance.

They claim that they just want to bring perspective to public health—to focus on real dangers, not imagined ones. Smoking kills 440,000 people a year in the United States alone, far more than any alleged toxin. They also make the controversial argument that millions worldwide have died of malaria because of the ban on the mosquito pesticide DDT. So DDT—which they claim poses a minimal threat to humans—should never have been outlawed.

"The chances of being sickened by any toxins is extremely slight," Seavey says. "There's no real risk, if any. It's a counterintuitive notion—the idea that something very bad for you could be harmless in small doses."

So why the obsession with toxins?

"It probably comes from our primitive caveman minds. We divide everything into either food or poison."

I agree with Seavey on that point. Putting aside which toxins are actually toxic, there's almost a religious element to the quest for purity from unnatural compounds. Toxin obsession reminds me of the intricate rules on kosher eating from when I lived by the Bible. Organic eaters look at chemicals the same way Orthodox Jews look at pork—as impure, almost repulsive.

There's this mistaken idea that natural is good, says Seavey. But arsenic and hemlock are natural. Likewise, there's the fallacious idea that natural products don't have chemicals. But they do. The ACSH claims on its website that "of the chemicals people eat, 99.99 percent are natural." Or as a wiseacre blogger wrote, "Even Rachel Carson was made of chemicals."

The Toxin-Free Life

Marti has e-mailed me a list of do's and don'ts for living a toxin-free life, I vow to spend the week following her path. Here are my notes for the first day:

9 a.m.: Trip to Whole Foods to buy organic strawberries and organic raspberries (price: $4.75). I can't listen to my

iPhone, per Marti, since she says it's linked to brain cancer and low sperm production. I'm bored out of mind.

10 a.m.: Morning ablutions. For my shower soap, I'm using olive oil mixed with mineral salts (got the recipe off an organic website). Felt very ancient Roman. For shampoo, baking soda and apple-cider vinegar. Took forever to wash it out, but my hair feels supersoft and has now has Einstein-like antigravity properties. Underarm deodorant is cornstarch and baking soda. Unpleasantly sticky.

11 a.m.: Cover Deca-laden upholstery on the couch with organic sheet.

Noon: Go on a BPA hunt in the kitchen, searching for the recycling code on the bottom of all plastic containers. Recite the classic BPA poem: "Four, five, one, and two/All the rest are bad for you."

1 p.m.: Explain to Julie why the couch is covered with organic sheet. Wait as she rolls her eyes.

2 p.m.: Meet friend Roger for a late lunch. He e-mails to ask for my cell. "I'm not carrying one these days. You can call the restaurant." He responds, "I'll send a Telex." Ha.

3 p.m.: Clean up spilled red wine in living room with vinegar and baking soda. Julie says this smells worse than spilled wine.

4 p.m.: I worry if the water bowl for our pet lizard, Brownie, contains BPA. I have the same thought about the plastic watering can for my plants. Realize this might not be best use of my cerebral cortex.

In short, I can't be as toxin-free as Marti. It's just not physically or logistically possible with three kids and all the other health-related things I have to do. But I don't want to glibly dismiss the dangers of toxins. There is lots of disturbing data out there—including that endocrine-related cancer has seen a 20 percent rise in the last ten years. There are 80,000 chemicals used in industrial processes, and only two hundred of them have been tested. What's the reasonable middle path?

I call up David Ewing Duncan, a journalist and public health advocate, who traced all the toxins in his body and wrote about it in his 2009 book *Experimental Man*.

How has his life changed after all the research?

"Many of the toxins I'm fatalistic about," he says. "Nobody knows how many parts per billion are dangerous. And even if we did, there's often nothing we can do about it. There's no way to escape. Virtually all the major chemicals are found everywhere on earth, from polar bears in the North Pole to penguins in the South Pole."

Are there things he does differently now that he's studied the issue for years?

"There are two behaviors I've changed."

First, he's much more careful about mercury in fish. He only eats sea creatures low on the food chain—crab and shrimp, for instance—which absorb less than the big predators, such as tuna and marlin.

Second, he says he'll never microwave anything in plastic again.

"But you could say I'm part of the problem, not the solution. There need to be people who are vigilant, like your aunt. We need to pay more attention before we add new chemicals."

It's all about weighing costs and benefits. To be totally safe, I could avoid cell phones. But the stress of living a cell-phone-free life? That might put me in an early grave. You have to choose your toxic battles.

I've made up a list for myself based on advice from toxicologists and the best available evidence, which I'm putting in the appendix.

Checkup: Month 12

Weight: 159 (how did it go up?)

Blood pressure: 100/69

Trips to gym this month: 15

Bottles of red wine consumed this year so far: 87

Bottles of dark red, antioxidant-rich Sardinian wine, which
supposedly helps the Sardinians' long life expectancy: 1

My current state of mind: self-righteous. I feared this would happen. I try to fight it, but I can feel it taking hold: I'm becoming a health fundamentalist.

I had the same experience when I lived by the Bible. After a few months, I became holier than thou, appalled by the sinfulness of the secular world. I'd flip through an *Us Weekly*, and curl my lip in disgust at all the coveting and greed and harlotry therein.

And now here I am, healthier than thou. I spend way too much time judging others. I know it's obnoxious, and probably unhealthy, but in my defense, I'm surrounded by some massive transgressions against the gods of health.

The other day, I watched a man on the street open a bag of Doritos. Apparently, he decided it would be too much effort to use his fingers to lift the triangular foodlike chips to his mouth. So he just shoved his face in the bag and started chomping away, like a horse with a feed bag. A while later, he came up for air, his face coated with glow-in-the-dark orange powder. I had to avert my eyes.

Later, I was running around the reservoir, and passed by two European tourists slowly walking and blowing smoke from their

Gitanes in the paths of runners. I turned around and glared at them the way the New England townspeople glared at Hester Prynne.

Sometimes my self-righteousness slips out. Julie was eating her Honey Bunches of Oats cereal this morning.

"How are your empty calories?" I asked.

"Delicious!" she said.

Then she added, "You're starting to sound like Marti."

She's got a point. Last time Marti was over, she told Jasper, who was drinking milk, "That's baby food. That's not meant for you, that's meant for baby cows. Baby food."

My self-righteousness is only reinforced by evidence that I may, in fact, be in good shape. Or at least in better shape than a major motion-picture action star.

My trainer Tony told me that Matt Damon works out at our gym. This is surprising, because it's not a fancy gym. There are plenty of gyms boasting varnished wooden lockers, coat-check girls, and cafés serving egg-white omelets. The gym I go to has a depressing Eastern European feel.

Tony says that Matt Damon comes into the gym a couple of days a week and works out for about half an hour till he's sweating and panting.

And here's the important part: His workout is *less* strenuous than mine. At least according to Tony, who says, "He wouldn't be able to do what you do. The jumping lunges alone would get him."

There's a chance Tony is saying this to make me feel better. There's also a chance Matt Damon is training for a role as an out-of-shape character, maybe for a biopic of Meat Loaf.

Still. It's exciting. I love bringing this information to Julie, who adopted Damon as her celebrity crush a few years ago after deeming Tom Cruise to be a nutter. "You like them apples?" I ask.

Chapter 13

The Teeth

The Quest for the Perfect Smile

I'VE BEEN PUTTING OFF DEALING with my teeth for months. Like four out of five consumers, I fear dentists. I also have empathy for dentists, mind you. It can't be fun being so loathed, to be the cod liver oil of the health care community.

But still I fear them. Perhaps it's because I got off to a bad start with tooth care. I had an orthodontist in fifth grade who, in his own way, was as sadistic as Laurence Olivier in *Marathon Man.* He'd sing me off-key Hebrew songs as I sat there, powerless to protest. He also had a cruel selection of magazines in his waiting room: Instead of *Highlights,* he had several copies of *Antiques* magazine so all the eleven-year-olds could marvel at the Townsend cabinets.

But I can't ignore my mouth forever. Because the annoying truth is, your teeth and gums are closely connected to the

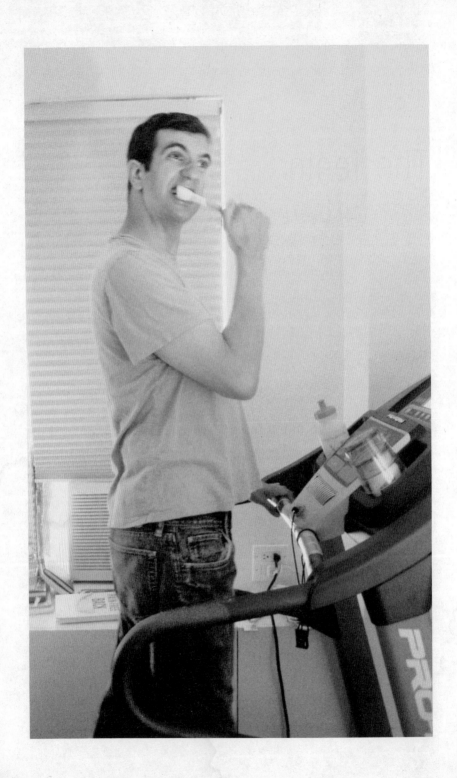

cardiovascular system. One study from Emory University found a significantly higher mortality rate—23 to 46 percent higher—among patients who suffered from periodontitis or gingivitis. Mouth bacteria—there are as many as a thousand types of it lurking in the cracks of your teeth—can seep into the blood and cause inflammation and hardening of the arteries.

Clean teeth are linked to a healthy heart. Their connection is why you get the scary—if not quite scientifically rock-solid—estimates that flossing will add 6.4 years to your life.

Right now I'm at a "dental spa." The Internet listed several and I figured I should try one. I didn't know what I'd find, but the word "spa" sounded so tranquil, I assumed it had to be an improvement in tooth care.

I thought perhaps it'd be a hushed oasis in midtown New York filled with the sound of bamboo wood chimes, the scent of citrus, and the sight of toned bodies. I'd slip on my complimentary fluffy white bathrobe and fluffy white slippers. I'd ease into a hot tub, maybe get a little seaweed wrap on my face. Then my spa dentist would massage my teeth with a lavender-scented loofah, not the mini-pickaxes used by regular nonspa dentists. Then I'd rinse my mouth with natural springwater from Baden Baden and leave in a state of joyful repose.

Instead, it turns out, a "dental spa" isn't too different from a "dental office."

Oh, they try to gussy it up a bit. There are purple-and-white crystals in the waiting room. A red Buddha figurine. And most spalike of all, I get a complimentary ten-minute foot massage. As I lie back, mouth ajar, with a dental hygienist jamming cotton into my cheeks, a bald man squeezes my toes and ankles. Not bad.

Still, there is no disguising that this is a dentist's office where unpleasant dental procedures take place. You can put patchouli oil on a pig, but it's still a pig.

Then again, maybe I should stop complaining. I just read an interesting and terrifying book called *The Excruciating History of Dentistry*. If you ever feel mopey about modern life—about how you can't get Wi-Fi in the train station, say—pick up this book. I don't have room to explain its horrible revelations, but consider these two facts: Dentists used to extract teeth with a large wrench while squeezing the writhing, unmedicated patient's head between the legs. And ancient Roman dentists prescribed tying a frog to the jaw as a way to fix loose teeth. So in comparison, a dental spa is paradise.

The dental spa offers the usual delights—fillings and root canals—but I'm here to get a regular old cleaning. And also to try a new procedure, or at least new for me: teeth whitening. CNN ran a story on my in-progress health quest, and I went ahead and read the comments on the Internet about the report. You know, just in case I was feeling too happy or secure. Some were nice, but I've blocked those out. The only one I remember: "He has yellow teeth, and he's trying to tell *me* how to be healthy?"

I wouldn't call them yellow. I prefer butter, oatmeal or eggshell, or something else more J.Crew catalog. But the commenter had a point. So off I went.

The dental hygienist—a bald, pudgy man—squirts bleach on my teeth, paints my lips with petroleum jelly, and inserts a large, blue rubber Hannibal Lecterish mouthpiece. Then he pulls the UV-light blasting machine down and sticks it against my teeth. I look like I'm kissing a DustBuster.

He explains that the UV light will activate the bleach and give me glowing teeth.

"Ishn't oo-vee light da-n-er-ous?" I ask.

He shakes his head. "No, no. This UV light is not dangerous."

He flips the switch, and the DustBuster starts humming. Forty-five minutes later, I look in the mirror. My teeth are definitely a few shades whiter. No one is going to mistake my mouth for an Antarctic snow drift, but they're better than before.

When I get home, I Google the safety of UV-light tooth-whitening treatments. Sure enough, it's not recommended. One study in a journal called *Photochemical & Photobiological Sciences* found that the treatments gave patients four times the radiation of sunbathing. Vanity can be dangerous.

String Theory and Practice

In the weeks preceding my dental spa appointment, I'd made several pilgrimages to a traditional, Western dentist and also interviewed an American Dental Association spokesperson. My question: How do I get the world's healthiest teeth? The answer is threefold, two-thirds of which are disappointing.

Let me get those out of the way first. Brushing and flossing. You can't avoid them.

Before this project, I'd flossed maybe three times in my life. I saw it as unnecessary, a bit show-offy. I brushed my teeth. Wasn't that enough? Sadly not. You need to clean your tooth cracks of the aforementioned thousand types of bacteria before they migrate to the bloodstream.

I started sharing Julie's Glide Comfort Plus floss. I do it each night before brushing (before is preferable, so that you can brush out the dislodged bacteria). Were you aware there's controversy over flossing methods? One faction recommends pulling the string all the way through the crack between each tooth so you don't cause damage when you tug the floss upward. I tried this. It took almost an extra scene of *30 Rock* to get through. So I've gone back to the slacker up-and-down method.

It's both amusing and depressing to me just how quickly I became self-righteous about my dental regimen. Just a month after I began flossing regularly, I had lunch with a friend who said she never stuck string between her teeth.

I looked at her dismissively. Then I heard myself saying: "How can you *not* floss?" Ah, the enthusiasm of the recent convert.

I also changed the way I brush. I got a soft toothbrush and pledged to scrub for two minutes. Two minutes! This is no small thing. Normally, I brush for twenty seconds. Two minutes requires Dalai Lama–level patience. It's best if you do those two minutes using what's called the modified Bass Method.

"Let me give you a lesson," I said to Julie one night in front of the bathroom mirror.

"Don't go up and down like you're erasing a pencil mark. Start at the gum at a forty-five-degree angle, and push the brush down. Then lift the brush back up to the gum and do it again."

She listened and tried it.

"Now that was actually helpful," she said.

"That's nice to hear."

"It's weird to realize you've been doing something wrong for forty years."

I know what she's saying. Before this project, I never knew I was doing so many everyday tasks incorrectly: chewing, going to the bathroom, brushing my teeth. Am I yawning properly? Sneezing? High schools should offer a class called Really Basic Life Skills 101.

And now for the third, far more pleasant part of tooth care: chewing gum.

Several studies have indicated that chewing sugar-free gum

after meals can help prevent tooth decay. This is especially true if the gum contains xylitol, a sweetener found in such brands as Ricochet, PowerBite, and some Trident products, because bacteria can't break it down. The Nordic nations are far ahead of us on this one. In Finland, schoolchildren are encouraged to chew xylitol gum.

Chewing gum provided a double thrill—unconsciously, I felt like I was doing something wrong, thanks to years of antigum propaganda from my parents. But intellectually, I knew I was doing something right.

Checkup: Month 13

Weight: 158

Total miles walked while writing: 810

Total hours spent watching *Dr. Oz* show: 156

Years closer to death: 1 (I had my birthday).

Sweet-potato fries stolen from my son's plate at various
   brunches: 36

I'm plugging away at my to-do list. Did I mention it's got lots of items? This month I was able to check off a big one: I attended a religious ritual, which is, at least arguably, good for the health.

We went to a Purim festival at our synagogue. Purim, as you might know, is the celebration of Queen Esther's rescue of the Jewish people from the evil King Ahasuerus. But over the centuries, it's evolved into a kind of Jewish Halloween. You dress up in costumes and eat high-fructose food.

It's preferable if the costumes have some sort of Jewish connection. My kids wore a Superman costume, a Batman costume, and a Flash costume.

I consoled myself that Superman is kind of Jewish. Like many Jews, he was an immigrant who changed his name. (Jules Feiffer calls Superman the "ultimate assimilationist fantasy.") Plus, he works in the media, which is a good Jewish thing to do.

In any case, we're off the temple.

"Come on, superheroes!" says Julie. "Let's get on those sneakers."

Let me take this moment to say that—as long as I don't eat the simple-carb-filled hamantaschen—this ritual is probably good for my health.

Numerous studies have shown that religion and health are linked. A study by the University of Texas's Population Research Center found that those who made weekly visits to a house of worship lived, on average, seven years longer than those who never visit.

As Stanford biologist Robert Sapolsky writes in *Why Zebras Don't Get Ulcers*, religion is thought to be healthy for several reasons, including:

- It provides a close-knit community.
- It gives a sense of purpose to life. Events happen for a reason—a worldview that lowers stress. If your child gets sick, you can say that God gave you this challenge because He knew you could handle it.

But before you go out and buy a stack of Bibles, let me toss in a whole bunch of caveats. As Sapolsky points out, studying religion's impact on health is tricky. There are tons of complicating factors. For one thing, some religious people might be less likely to smoke or drink heavily. Plus, he says, "Religion can be very good at reducing stressors, but it is often the inventor of those stressors in the first place." If you believe that masturbation will land you in hell, your cortisol will rise.

In any case, there's at least some correlation between religion and health. Which isn't exactly why we joined the synagogue. Julie and I joined this synagogue after my year of living biblically because we wanted to give our sons a taste of their heritage, even if they decide to ignore it later.

I won't, unfortunately, get the stress-reducing benefit of believing that everything was meant to happen for a divine reason. I'm agnostic. Or more precisely, after my year of living biblically, I'm an agnostic with a veneration for rituals. As a pastor friend calls it, I'm a "reverent agnostic." Whether or not there's a God, I feel there's room for the sacred in my life. Prayers of thanksgiving can be sacred. Time with the family can be sacred. Dressing up as Superman—definitely sacred.

And the Sabbath—that can be sacred as well. I still try to observe the Sabbath. I don't do the full Orthodox no-pressing-elevator-buttons Shabbat. I just try not to answer my e-mails or do Facebook updates, and try to spend the day with my family.

This year, I've had to grapple with whether to exercise on the Sabbath, since for me, exercise *is* work. I figure running after my kids as they zoom down the sidewalk on their Razor scooters? That's okay. Going to the gym? I try to avoid it.

There haven't been a lot of rigorous studies on whether the Sabbath reduces stress, but I do know that I get a feeling of release on Friday night, a school's-out-for-summer wave of relief.

We arrived at the synagogue and went downstairs. Dozens of Spider Mans and princesses and a couple of Scooby-Doos scampered around the synagogue basement. The kids flipped the stuffed frogs into the holes in a carnival game. Zane gets a smiley face painted on his cheek by a middle school volunteer. He'll later cry about spilled toothpaste, and the his tears will smear the smiley face, an irony that even he, a four-year-old, had to admit was kind of amusing. But overall, it's good to be a part of this community, any community, and my cortisol levels recede.

Chapter 14

The Feet

The Quest to Run Right

I AM IN A CHAIN of sixty people, a sort of conga line without the Gloria Estefan music. Hands on one another's shoulders, we are snaking our way through a park in Harlem.

About half of the human chain wears no shoes. Many other feet are encased snugly in red or yellow or black Vibram FiveFingers shoes—those gloves for the feet that my kids call "monkey shoes." Others have fashioned their own footwear. Two college-age guys have taken flat rubber soles, attached leather straps, and entwined them gladiator-style around their calves.

I'm here at the meeting place for the first annual Barefoot Run in New York, led by the high priest of shoeless jogging, Christopher McDougall, author of *Born to Run.*

We will soon set out across Manhattan, but first we are warming up by pattering around Marcus Garvey Park. The organizers have

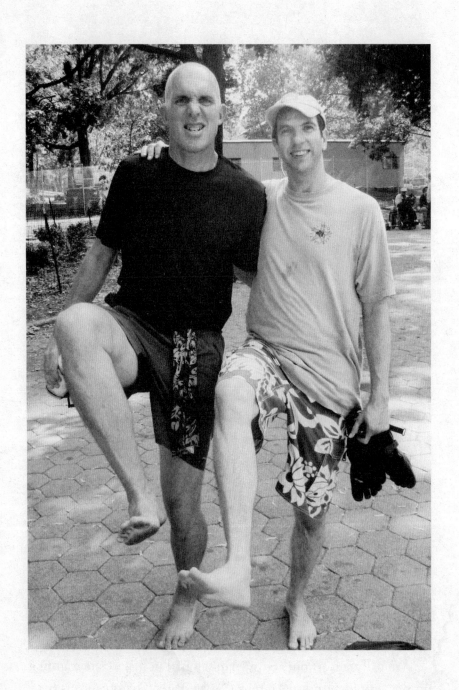

hired two guys in tracksuits to thump African drums to get us in the barefoot-running mood before we head downtown. Not that this herd of runners need it, really. They are already converts.

The conversations revolve around the time they saw the light. That moment they revolted against the footwear industry, and threw off their well-padded, overengineered lace-up chains. "I just said F it, and took off my shoes!" recounts a woman in red shorts. They talk about their freedom from plantar warts and aching arches.

I'm working on my feet this month because they are a huge, and often overlooked, health hazard. Americans suffer an estimated nine million foot injuries a year. And as I get older, I can look forward to more and more malfunctions. They take a beating, those feet. Even a lazy American still walks the equivalent of the earth's circumference in his or her lifetime.

I spot McDougall. He's a tall man with his Vibrams tucked into waistband of his forest-green shorts. A purple do-rag covers his bald head.

I introduce myself. He's warm and welcoming—and just as surprised as anyone that his "niche book," as he calls it, blew up and started a movement. It has sold nearly a million copies. The idea of the 2009 tome is simple. Our feet evolved to run barefoot, which is what humans have been doing for thousands of years. Then along came these foot prisons called shoes. In the 1970s, Nike made everything worse with their fixation on soft padding. Instead of preventing injuries—which is what sneakers promised—they actually caused them. They encouraged us to land hard on the heel, putting stress on the knees and the shins. McDougall's ideal runners are a tribe in Mexico's Copper Canyons called the Tarahumara, who wear slender pieces of rubber strapped to their feet.

I bought Vibrams a few months ago. When I brought them home, Julie and the boys had a nice belly laugh at the way they looked on my feet.

"Poor Ashton Kutcher. He can't wear them," Julie said, showing me a line in the manual that says Vibrams won't fit on webbed feet. Apparently, Kutcher has webbed feet. My wife's knowledge of pop culture knows no bounds.

I took a couple of runs in them. I haven't yet decided on whether I prefer them to sneakers. The Vibrams have their advantages: The rubber is so thin, you feel like you're jogging around New York in bare feet. You can make out the contours of the curb with your toes. Which is a liberating and hilarious, an almost naughty sensation. Bare feet! In the city. It's like Columbus Avenue has merged with your bedroom, or has magically transformed into a Caribbean beach. And so far, no rusty nails or blisters.

I'm wearing my Vibrams for today's run. I wish I could have gone full McDougall, but I'm germaphobic, and fear contact between my naked soles and the sidewalk, so Vibrams it is.

McDougall gathers us round to give us a primer on technique. We're told to land lightly on the front of the foot and let the heels just kiss the ground.

Take small steps. Cushy sneakers encourage long strides because the heels don't hurt as they pound the ground. But that's not what humans are meant to do. And also, try to pull your legs up instead of stomping them down.

"Think of it like you have pancakes on your upper thighs, and you're trying to raise your knees to flip them," McDougall says.

And perhaps, most important, it's about being joyful when you run.

And with that, off we go. We trot west on 125th Street, past shops and street vendors selling Bob Marley posters. We look a little odd, flipping our imaginary pancakes, and we do not go unnoticed by the pedestrians.

"Put on some damn shoes!"

"Stop running like a bunch of girls!" (The toe-first running does have a certain prancing tenor to it.)

"White people are taking over Harlem!"

We enter the park and head up a gentle hill, making our way toward the reservoir. I catch up with McDougall, and we pat along.

"Look at this," he says, stopping and showing me the bottom of his foot. It's midnight black.

"Do you worry about stepping on things?" I huff.

"It doesn't bother me. I live in rural Pennsylvania, so I step in all sorts of things. Horseshit, you name it. You learn to avoid the sharp objects," he says.

I ask him to critique my running.

"You've got a heel-heavy stride, man!"

I land too hard on the back of my foot. I try leaning forward more. "That's better." McDougall says.

I tell him that I sometimes run on the treadmill at the gym, which I suspect he thinks is a bad idea. I'm right.

"You tend to want to race the treadmill, so you take big strides," he says. "If you have to do it, my advice would be to go right up to the front of the treadmill, so your hips are right against the bars. Not to get too carnal about it, but get up there and go at it." He mimes a dry hump. It may seem lascivious, McDougall says, but I'll be taking smaller steps.

McDougall trots off to help another runner. A few minutes later, we're running down a Central Park path, all sixty of us, when we see a stocky jogger heading right toward us.

He grimaces as he tries to navigate his way through this river of half-barefoot people.

"Oh, come on!" he shouts as he brushes by us.

"Wow, he seemed angry," I say.

"I think it's because he was wearing shoes," says a barefoot woman.

We laugh.

"They were probably too tight and giving him bad energy."

"He's like the Grinch. His shoes are two sizes too small," calls out another runner.

I love being an insider, a member of the shoeless Mafia. Those poor squares trapped in their sneaker jails. But as for the pure joy of running that McDougall speaks about? I'm not feeling it.

The Appropriately Named Foot Doctor

A couple of weeks later, I ended up in the office of Dr. Krista Archer. Dr. Archer is a respected foot surgeon in New York with shoulder-length blond hair. She often appears on morning TV to talk about, say, how to minimize damage from stiletto heels.

I'd come to see her for some advice on how to have the healthiest feet, and also to get her take on the great barefoot debate.

Should I exercise without shoes?

"I'm not an advocate," she says.

She explains: If you have no foot problems, if your feet are models of biomechanical perfection, going shoeless might be fine. But if you have any quirks, if, for instance, your foot rolls inward or outward too much, then put on the sneakers.

"Running puts a huge load on the feet—three times the body weight on the front foot."

But isn't the foot designed to run barefoot? "That doesn't mean it's the best way to do it," Dr. Archer says. "We used to use dial-up modems. Should we stick with them? If you're nearsighted, should you avoid glasses because they're not 'natural'?"

In fact, she suggests that I buy a foam insert for my sneakers. As McDougall said, I do land too hard on my heels.

I'll return to Dr. Archer in a moment, but let me say this. After talking to other doctors and reading everything I could on the topic, I can confidently say: The jury's still out on the barefoot movement. It shouldn't be dismissed as a wackadoodle fad. It does make some logical sense. But on the other hand, it probably shouldn't be adopted by everyone. Medicine is increasingly personal, and the feet are no exception. It's something to try. Nowadays, I take about a quarter of my runs sans shoes.

Back in Dr. Archer's office, I slip off my shoes and socks for my exam.

She looks at my heels, which are covered in thick, callused skin. They have cracks big enough to fit dimes, maybe nickels.

Her diagnosis: "Ouchy."

I'm going to need to add another task to my enormous list of daily commandments: exfoliating my heels in the shower. I tell her she should have seen my feet a week ago. Julie just took me to my first pedicure as part of Project Health, and the Korean woman spent five minutes polishing my heel.

"Did you like the pedicure?" she asked.

"Not really," I say. The whole woman-kneeling-at-your-feet dynamic made me feel too much like a viceroy of a British colony.

"You have to be careful with pedicures," she says.

Dr. Archer lists all the horrible problems that pedicures can unleash. When you get a pedicure, she tells me, you are submerging your feet in a swamp of germs. The jets in the footbath are clogged with bits of skin from previous clients.

"People get fungus all the time from pedicures," she says.

If I ever go again, she says, I should bring my own nail file, clippers, and buffers. In fact, Archer is releasing an antifungal treatment—it's made from tea tree oil—that I could apply to my toes pre- and post-pedicure.

"And you should never let them cut the cuticles," she says. "The cuticles are your body's defense against bacteria." I assure her, my cuticles will remain intact.

Checkup: Month 14

Weight: 157

New vocabulary words learned to keep brain in shape: 301

    (Today's: "*cyanosis*," the condition of having blue skin.)

Quinoa consumed since start of project: 44 pounds

Pounds lifted on squat machine (15 reps): 360

I'm typing this update in a tiny rented basement office. To get work done, I needed a refuge from my lovable but boundary-defying children.

It's a depressing and dank little dungeon that's only missing the foot chains. The upside? It's freezing. At times, I have to put on my Patagonia overcoat and type with a pair of fingerless gloves.

This is good, because being cold burns more calories. A 2009 article in the journal *Obesity Reviews* by a University College London professor reports that the obesity epidemic can be blamed partly on our tendency to crank up the thermostat. American bedroom temperature has crept up from 66.7 degrees in 1987 to 68 in 2005. When it's chilly, we have to burn more fuel just to maintain our body temperature. Cold also activates something called brown fat, which is easier to burn than white fat.

My friend Tim Ferriss's book *The 4-Hour Body* recommends cold therapy for weight loss. He says an ice pack on the back of the neck will help. Or if you're a tough guy, a ten-minute ice bath. I hate that my dungeon has no treadmill desk, but at least I am shivering.

Incidentally, my arctic conditions haven't given me a cold. Which makes sense, since even Ben Franklin pointed out more than two centuries ago that cold doesn't cause colds.

But everyone else in my family does have a cold. Lucas, Zane, Jasper, Julie—they're all sneezing and wheezing. I'm the only one in no need of a neti pot.

It's no fun to be surrounded by cranky coughers, and I feel terrible, especially for Lucas, who is leaking like the maddening air conditioner on the floor above us. But there's a small part of me that is smugly satisfied.

All this sweating, eating right, and stressing less—maybe it's working. Maybe this is what it feels like to be healthy. Maybe my overly welcoming immune system has finally decided to get rude. It's a historic time.

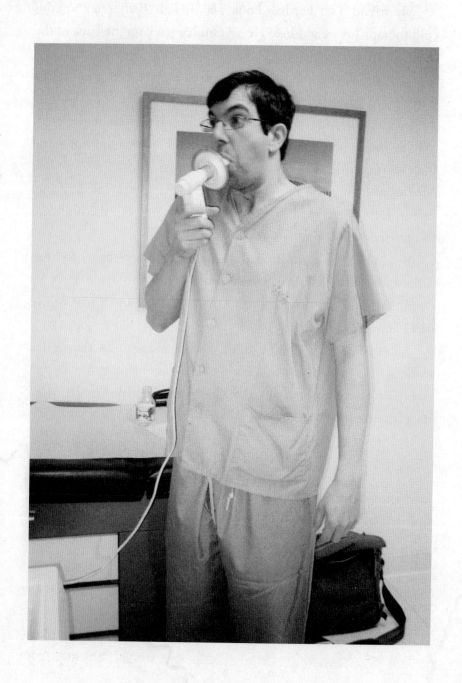

Chapter 15

The Lungs

The Quest to Breathe Better

THE SATURDAY, we take our kids to the *Bodies* exhibit at South Street Seaport. This popular museum exhibit displays actual cadavers in various positions. Some are cut into delilike slices. Some are stripped of skin and frozen in heroic stances, such as tossing a football or conducting a symphony.

The exhibit is a little more graphic than I anticipated. Maybe a little much for my four-year-old twins. Maybe a little much for me. In the bone section, one glass case holds a tiny pelvic bone from what looks to be a six-month-old child.

The woman next to me peers into the glass case, spots the remains, and says, with all earnestness, "Ohhhh. That's so cute." To me, not cute. Harrowing. It reminds me of Casper the Friendly Ghost, the strangest comic book in history. The creators just gloss right over the horrid backstory. Are we just supposed to forget that a child had to die to produce this chipper poltergeist?

Luckily, my sons aren't too fazed. They are most interested by a huge plastic container filled waist-high with packs of discarded cigarettes. They love the colors and designs on the boxes.

A sign next to the container warns: EVERY TIME YOU SMOKE A PACK OF CIGARETTES, YOU LOSE THREE HOURS AND FORTY MINUTES OFF YOUR LIFE. Passersby are encouraged to drop their packs in the slot and regain those hours.

"Why do people smoke?" Jasper asks as we walk to the next room.

"Well, you know how Zane liked his pacifier?" Julie says. "It's the same thing with grown-ups and cigarettes. It feels good. It gives you something to do with the mouth. Also, they're supposed to be relaxing."

What is she saying? Maybe she should add that cigarettes have a cool, refreshing flavor, like you're breathing Rocky Mountain air.

I shoot her a look. "You don't have to sell it quite that hard."

"Yeah, that didn't come out right," she says.

For someone who hates smoking as much as Julie, she sure knows how to talk it up. If we find Parliaments in our boys' Incredible Hulk backpacks, I'll know whom to blame.

I've been focusing on my lungs this month. Without those eleven-pound organs—and their 1,500 miles of airways and 500 million tiny air sacs—I wouldn't be around to worry about any other body parts.

I've been reading a lot about smoking. I almost wish I'd been a smoker. That way, I could have made a huge improvement by quitting during Project Health. But sadly, I smoked my only cigarette at age fifteen. I spent the next ten minutes getting sick while clutching a sidewalk trash can with both hands.

So cigarettes made me ill in the short run. Which saved me from getting ill in the long run. Cigarettes are still the leading preventable cause of death in America, killing about 440,000 people a year. The unfortunate part is, if they weren't so horribly bad for you, cigarettes could be very handy in stopping the obesity epidemic. Nicotine is one of the only proven appetite suppressants. Studies show that smokers are generally thinner than us nonpuffers. The cigarette industry has tried to exploit the weight-loss angle over the years. Consider the cleverly named Virginia Slims brand that was marketed to women. Or else Lucky's famous 1920s campaign of "reach for a Lucky instead of a sweet." (Which incidentally, spawned one of the most ridiculous feuds in health history: The National Confectioners Association threatened to sue Lucky. The candy lobby published antismoking pamphlets that, as Allan Brandt writes in *The Cigarette Century*, stressed the importance of candy as food.)

But alas, cigarettes' costs far outweigh any resulting trimness, just as asphyxiation outweighs the benefits of stretching out the spine when you hang yourself from a shower curtain rod.

The Science of Inhaling and Exhaling

I've been breathing wrong my whole life. By my calculations, I've taken 220,752,000 incorrect breaths, plus or minus.

According to people who think about the lungs a lot, my problem is twofold: I breathe shallowly and through my mouth.

Let me take those problems one at a time.

I've always been a mouth breather. When I listen back to interviews I've tape-recorded, it sounds like Darth Vader is doing push-ups in the background. I'd hoped this year to learn that mouth breathing is good for you, so I could proclaim its benefits and start a Mouth Breathing Pride movement.

Sadly, it's not. The nose conditions the air—it warms it up, humidifies it, and filters out harmful bacteria. It provides multiple lines of defense, including regular hair, microscopic hair (cilia), bones called turbinates, and mucus. Plus, some doctors argue that nose breathing produces nitrous oxide, which dilates the blood vessels and increases oxygen absorption.

And then there's deep breathing. According to Dr. Andrew Weil, the mostly nonquacky alternative health guru, deep breathing "slows your heart rate, lowers blood pressure and improves circulation."

I decided I needed some lessons in deep breathing. First, I went to see the owner of perhaps the most famous pair of lungs in America—David Blaine. Blaine has the world record for holding his breath. He did it for seventeen minutes and four seconds. He used a method called "lung-packing," where you breathe in as much air as you can, then squeeze in even more air with four short inhalations, (I know this is an overused phrase, but if there's one time it fits, this is it: PLEASE do not do this at home.)

I'd met Blaine when I interviewed him for *Esquire*. I went into the article skeptically, but found him charming and thoughtful. Plus, he's obsessed with health. (His morning juice recipe, which I've tested several times: "Two cloves of garlic, bok choy, kale, collard greens, spinach, half a beet, half an apple, two lemons, and cayenne pepper.")

I arrived at Blaine's office, with its huge posters of Houdini and a motorcycle in the entryway. When I got there, Blaine was on the phone having a normal, everyday conversation about an upcoming appearance. "Yeah, this is the last time I'm going to eat glass," he says. "I promised my fiancée. It does crazy damage. It rips up my stomach, takes all the enamel off my teeth." Agreed. Blaine hangs up.

He offers me a fist-sized stalk of raw ginger, supposedly good for preventing colon cancer and inflammation. It would be rude to say no.

"Just chew it, get the juice, then spit it out," he says. He tears into a hunk of his own with his enamel-free teeth.

I ask him about what to do to get the healthiest lungs.

"If you want the cleanest air, you should move to Tasmania or Antarctica. But if that's not possible, you should get an IQAir Purifier. It's the brand that the athletes used in the Beijing Olympics."

And what about deep breathing? I don't need to hold my breath for a quarter of an hour. But I would like to breathe deeper.

Blaine inhales. "Feel the air fill your lungs," he says. I do. "Now feel the air fill your stomach, your shoulders, everywhere." I try to imagine my whole torso filling with air. I hold it in, and then exhale. Blaine doesn't.

"Now let's do some stretches," he says.

"How do you like your ginger?" he asks as we slowly wave our arms overhead. I tell him it's got more of a kick than I imagined. He still hasn't exhaled.

Before I leave, we chat some more about the *Esquire* article. He does, eventually, exhale. I liked Blaine's advice about trying to get air into every crevice of your upper body. But I wanted a second opinion.

I got it from a vocal coach named Justin Stoney. Stoney had me lie on the floor, put my hand on my stomach, and feel it rise when I inhaled. "Don't even try to inhale," he said. "Just push out your stomach, and you'll create a vacuum, and the air will come in. When you exhale, flatten your stomach out."

This stomach-breathing turned out to be a life changer. A small life changer, but still. When I run, I stomach-breathe, and I don't do nearly as much huffing and puffing as I used to. It saves me from that unpleasant burning-chest feeling. I'm doing it right now, at my treadmill desk. I'm pushing out my stomach on the inhale so that it resembles an Al Gore–like potbelly, then sucking back in on the exhale.

Moments of Zen

I can't leave the topic of deep breathing without mentioning meditation. Meditation, like yoga and libertarianism, has gone mainstream. Marines meditate cross-legged, their rifles on their laps, as part of their training. My six-year-old son does breathing exercises at school (though their mantra is the not-so-Hindi "sniff the flower, blow out the candle"). The medical benefits are rock-solid: lower rates of depression and heart disease, improved attention.

I first learned meditation from a Zen center in the Village when I wrote an article on unitasking—the art of only doing one thing at a time. For the past few months, I've been meditating a couple of times a week in the living room, after Julie's gone to sleep, sitting on the floor and staring at the wall for ten minutes.

But lately, I've tried to meditate every day. Because of time constraints, I end up doing what I call contextual meditation. I meditate anywhere when I have five minutes—on the bus, on the subway, waiting for a walk sign.

I'm not alone. I found a wellness website with instructions on how to meditate in a noisy environment. I tried it when I was undergoing an MRI the other day (I was getting scanned for a brief episode of blurry vision, which turned out to be nothing.) Now, if you've never had an MRI, you should know that they are loud, almost comically so. The technician gives you earplugs, but that doesn't come close to blocking the sound. The MRI has a repertoire of noises that resemble, in no particular order: game-show buzzer for a wrong answer, urgent knocking, a modem from 1992, a grizzly-bear growl, and a man with a raspy voice shouting what sounds like "mother cooler!"

The key is to let the noise glide through your brain without stopping to interpret it. Don't try to block out the sound waves. Just notice them as they float by, and say, "Isn't that interesting." The website tells us not to ponder the sounds' origins. Instead focus on the tones and vibrations. "Mo-ther-coo-ler. Mo-ther-coo-ler."

That's quite a sound. But it doesn't bother me. It was the most relaxing MRI of my life.

A Breath of Fresh Air

On a Wednesday for lunch, Julie and I go to visit my grandfather. He is, no surprise, stretched out on the recliner, wearing a red shirt with long sleeves. He looks older. His wrists are as thin as broomstick handles, his eyes rheumy. His breathing is labored. Which is understandable. As you age, the lungs deteriorate. They lose the air sacs and capillaries, the diaphragm weakens, the muscles get less elastic.

Julie leans down to kiss him.

"Hi, dear," he says, in between breaths.

He asks about my boys, but I can tell he can't remember their names.

"What are you working on, A.J.?" he asks.

I tell him I am writing about lungs. "You know, you helped New Yorkers' lungs," I say.

"Oh?" he says.

"All the mass transit projects you worked on. You helped cut down on pollution."

"Oh, yes?"

He seems pleased, but confused. I remind him of his bold idea. Long a booster of the subway and bus system, my grandfather decided a couple of years ago that mass transit should be free, like water or radio. The result would be fewer people driving cars, less smog, more efficiency. He funded a study and lobbied the mayor.

"That's going to happen soon," he says. Typical optimism, perhaps delusional.

"Hope so," I say.

New York's air pollution is bad, but it could be much worse. The American Lung Association recently found it to be the sixteenth worst city for ozone pollution (Bakersfield, California, got first) and the twenty-first for particle pollution (Los Angeles won the title).

Air pollution causes all sorts of problems, including emphysema, asthma, and cardiac diseases. The World Health Organization estimates that 2.1 million people die from air-pollution-related diseases every year. But that's just a rough guess. It's unclear how many New Yorkers succumb.

The best you can do is try to keep your house's air clean. Don't use scented candles or products. Clean the air conditioner every year. Some doctors say you should open the windows for fifteen minutes a day, because indoor air tends to be dirtier than outdoor air. If you have lung problems, buy a HEPA filter. And if you're *really* committed, buy an N95 surgical mask, a special kind that screens out particles. I tested one out while walking on my smelly, rubber-burning treadmill. It was rain-forest hot to breathe into it.

"You seem to have survived the pollution, Grandpa," Julie points out.

"Still hanging in there," he replies, smiling.

"Actually, you picked a good place to live, Grandpa," I say.

I tell him that despite the pollution, New York has a surprisingly high life expectancy: 78.6 as opposed to the national average of 77.8. Why? Theories vary, but most agree that a lot of it has to do with the amount New Yorkers walk. As the city's former commissioner of public health told *New York* magazine, New York is like one big gym.

"Though you could have done a little better," I say. "Like Okinawa."

The southern Japanese prefecture has the highest number of centenarians, thanks to a mix of factors (steep hills for walking, lots of manual labor even among the elderly, a low-fat, high-carb, low-sugar diet, etc.).

"Or you could have been a Seventh Day Adventist in San Diego." Another cluster of extremely long-lived people, thanks in part to close family ties and a strict no-meat diet.

"The what now?" he says.

"Seventh Day Adventists. They're a religious group. You could join."

"I think it's too late."

Checkup: Month 15

Weight: 158

Packs of gum chewed since tooth chapter: 48

Minutes spent meditating per day: 10

Minutes of that when actually meditating as opposed to
 thinking of something trivial: 2

My sedentary behavior is down to about four hours a day. Have I mentioned how much I love walking on the treadmill? I type on it, brush my teeth on it, take my fish-oil supplements on it. It gives me a sense of accomplishment, as odd as that may sound for something designed to keep you in place. I've now been working on this book for 880 miles. I'm hoping to break a thousand by the end.

I often wonder what the previous me would think of the me that I've become. I'm now the guy who wears bike shorts even when not biking. I'm the only one at parties who actually eats the crudités. At restaurants, I ask if the salmon is farm-raised or wild. And that it not be blackened (blackening has been linked to cancer). And that there be no starch on the plate when it is served.

I think the previous me would avoid me.

Chapter 16

The Stomach, Revisited

The Continued Quest for the Perfect Diet

I'M EATING A LOT OF the same foods every day, which I'm not sure is such a good idea. Here's my daily menu for the last month or so:

Breakfast: two scrambled egg whites in canola oil, a handful
  of walnuts, a bowl of steel-cut oatmeal topped with organic
  blueberries, strawberries, and flaxseed oil.
Lunch: chopped salad of spinach, broccoli, red cabbage,
  mixed peppers, peas, tomatoes, avocado, artichoke hearts,
  beets, and (sometimes) sunflower seeds. No dressing.
Afternoon snack: fat-free Greek yogurt with cantaloupe and
  grapes. Three spoonfuls of hummus.
Dinner: quinoa, steamed asparagus, Dr. Praeger's spinach
  pancake. And three times a week, grilled wild salmon with
  lemon juice (sorry, Marti). Glass of red wine. Maybe two.

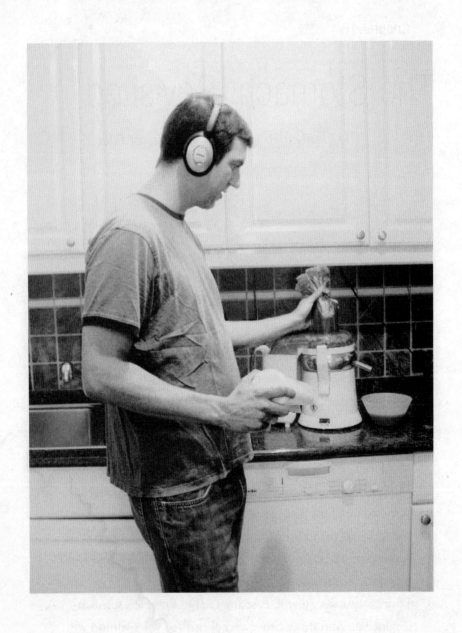

It's basically a modified Mediterranean diet, the diet that is perhaps supported by the most studies. I don't mind the sameness. It's my comfort food. But for the sake of health, I should probably mix it up more. Do something crazy, like substitute bulgur for quinoa.

And for the sake of self-experimentation, I should go to the extremes. I should road-test some of the diets I've been reading about. For the next few weeks, I pledge to sample the two poles of the nutrition world: the raw-food vegan diet and the Paleo-Atkins-type diet.

Raw Food

My aunt Marti is in town, and we meet at a vegan restaurant on the East Side called Candle 79. I've asked Marti to give me a personal *Idiot's Guide* to raw foodism.

We sit down in the back corner. Marti doesn't like the toxins emitted by the eponymous candles. She asks that the one on our table be removed.

"It's not a real candle," says the waitress. "It's electric."

"I'd still like it taken away—the electromagnetic pollution."

With the candle gone, I ask Marti's advice on going raw. "You're going to have to get over your aversion to making your own food," she tells me.

I need to get: a blender, a slicer, a spiralizer, a dehydrator, spirulina powder, blue-green algae crystals, and Himalayan or Celtic sea salt. I need a juicer, but not just any juicer—I need it with an auger gear, not a centrifuge, since the blades oxidize the food and lower its nutritional value.

Oh man. As I scribble my notes, I feel my book advance slowly slipping away.

My auger-geared juicer arrived a couple of days later. Within an hour I had baptized it in blood from my ring finger, which I accidentally sliced while fitting the parts together.

I took out my plastic bags of organic cucumbers, kale, carrots, beets, Swiss chard, and zucchini. I put the zucchini into the juicer and pushed down. Nothing. I pushed harder. A whirring and thumping as the juicer devoured the zucchini and leaked out a weak green stream on the other end. That's right. I'm juicing!

After decimating several vegetables, I decide juicing is my favorite form of food preparation. There's something perversely appealing about subjecting an innocent plant to that much violence. It's the closest I'll ever get to hunting.

The juicing takes forty-five minutes, much of that time devoted to rinsing the myriad parts. As Marti warned, raw food is astoundingly time-consuming. You'd think not cooking would be a time-saver. You would be wrong.

And juicing is microwave-quick compared to another noncooking technique: dehydrating. My dehydrator was delivered the other day—a black box the size of an air conditioner, with removable shelves. In raw food circles, you're forbidden from using heat higher than 104° F. because it supposedly destroys the living enzymes. So the dehydrator blows warm air on your food for hours, sometimes days. It reminds me of the temperature and intensity of dog's breath. So imagine a German shepherd exhaling on your fruit for a day. I dried apples, oranges, carrots, strawberries, and blueberries into chewy leathery slices. Not bad, the family agreed. Dehydrating is glacial, but at least it's hard to screw up.

After two weeks of juicing and dehydrating, here's my assessment:

Positive: I feel lighter and cleaner. And I discovered that raw food, if prepared properly, can be tasty. I've spent hours on raw food websites downloading recipes (and studying raw food humor: "You know you are a raw vegan when your pots and pans are the new fruit baskets). The avocado-and-mango salad? Zesty goodness.

Negative: I am hungry all the time, and I started to look gaunt. "What's with the manorexic look?" my friend asked. By the end, I'd lost three pounds. (So, if weight loss is your goal, raw food is something to consider.) In other news, it made me feel light-headed and spacey. Also, since you asked, it was the most flatulent two weeks of my life. I was tempted to call Dr. Gottesman for some surgery.

Marti will kill me for saying so, but the mainstream scientific evidence for the raw food diet isn't overly strong. There's lots of evidence in favor of a plant-based diet, but the raw part is less established. If done properly, with enough protein and B12 supplements, it's certainly better than the Standard American Diet. (Then again, eating nothing but asbestos sandwiches is probably better than the Standard American Diet.)

The War on Carbs

On the other side of the spectrum we find the low-carb, high-protein diets, such as the Atkins and the Paleo regimes. Before embarking on one, I asked John Durant—the reasonable caveman from the wilderness workout—if he'd answer my questions. He suggested we meet at a Korean barbecue restaurant in midtown.

At a Korean barbecue, in case you've never been, you get to cook your own food over a Frisbee-size grill in the middle of your table. Fire and meat. It's all quite Stone Age, except for the waiters, sparkling water, and gender-separated bathrooms.

Durant is a good-looking caveman, with long hair he sometimes ties in a ponytail and a tidily trimmed beard. Durant works at an Internet start-up, a job he will later quit to become, as he put it, a "professional caveman," and devote his time to writing a book.

He appeared on *The Colbert Report*, where he joked that his ideal girlfriend would have celiac disease and be unable to eat grains. Forty women with grain allergies e-mailed him after the show.

The waiter approaches. Durant orders some cow intestine. I go with the fish and vegetables.

I ask him if he ever eats raw meat, like Vlad does.

"I eat raw meat in socially acceptable ways," Durant says. "There are a surprising number of ways—sushi, sashimi, steak tartare."

At home, Durant has a three-foot-tall refrigerated meat locker with organ meat and deer ribs. But that's only part of his diet.

"There's a misconception that we only eat meat off rib bones. We eat a lot of vegetables and eggs and some nuts." The idea is to avoid dairy, grass seeds, potatoes, and grain, which were developed only in the last ten thousand years.

How does the Paleo diet make him feel?

"Much better. My complexion is better. I don't get mood spikes like I used to. I've lost twenty to twenty-five pounds."

The Paleo diet made me feel amazingly full. Protein and fats are the most satiating types of food. This why the low-carb diets can be so effective when it comes to weight loss—your body produces less insulin, which often translates to dampened hunger.

I must confess, Durant might not have approved of some of my choices. The first night, I tried veal, but it was like a drone strike in my stomach. Plus, my aunt Marti's decades-long campaign instills guilt in me when I eat mammals. I switched my protein intake to eggs, fish, and nuts. Still, I noticed a jump in energy, much less of my usual afternoon lethargy.

As with raw food, the evidence for the Paleo diet is still inconclusive. It probably helps you lose weight if you're obese, as do most carb-restricting diets. But it's not clear what effect the diet has on heart disease. We also don't know if this is actually the diet that our ancestors ate. Paleo skeptics—such as Marion Nestle—point out that plants from prehistoric kitchens wouldn't leave fossils.

The Not So Dolce Vita

I conduct one other dietary experiment: living a sugar-free life.

Sugar has never been a favorite of dieticians, parents, or dentists. But now its reputation is in a steep descent, challenging tobacco as Public Health Enemy number one. The sugar-is-toxic movement has taken wing thanks to two convincing publicizers, Dr. Robert Lustig, a professor of pediatrics at UCSF, and Gary Taubes, the science writer. The argument is that sugar in any form—white table sugar, high-fructose corn syrup, fruit juice—isn't just empty calories. Sugar wreaks havoc on your liver and pancreas, and makes cells resistant to insulin, which leads to diabetes and obesity. In the language of bumper stickers, SUGAR-DEATH.

There are plenty of sugar defenders out there. Sugar is fine in moderation, they say. One doctor, David Katz of the Yale Prevention Research Center, points out that sugar is the hummingbird's sole source of energy: "How evil can hummingbird fuel be?"

Pretty evil, the hard-core sugar haters say. They advise avoiding fruit high on the sweetness scale (pineapple and watermelon, for instance), and even suggest drinking low-sugar wine like Sauvignon Blanc instead of Chardonnay. They point out studies that show that sugar is addictive. It has the same effect on the brain as cocaine.

My favorite depressing fact is that just *thinking* about it—sugar might be bad for you. Taubes writes that the sweet thoughts trigger a Pavlovian response that includes saliva, gastric juices, and, most unhealthily, the release of insulin. So to be truly healthy, I should refuse to watch *Willy Wonka and the Chocolate Factory* with my kids.

As always in nutrition, the sugar debate is a big old murky mess of evidence. But I do think there's a good chance that sugar is a lot worse than we've long thought. So I'm going to give it up for at least two weeks. No juices, no granola, nothing with the dreaded suffix "ose."

This self-imposed Lent will be hard. When I talk to Taubes, he suggests the out-of-sight-out-of-mind strategy is probably best. Remove all sweets from the house. "Total abstention from refined carbs and sweets—losing your sweet tooth—may be ultimately easier than trying to eat them in moderation." But Taubes has young kids, so that won't be happening in his life. Nor mine.

Consider dried mangoes. My kids are allowed to eat a couple of slices after lunch. But I'm addicted to them as well, polishing off as many as twenty in a day.

Dried mangoes have the veneer of healthiness—which is why I originally chose them as our treat of choice. But really, they're just Snickers that happen to grow on trees. Those mango slices are delivering sixty grams of sugar to my blood each day—the equivalent of fifteen teaspoons of white sugar.

My willpower is failing me here. I've tried several strategies to kick this mango habit. I put them as far away from eye level as possible, tucking them behind a tray on the top shelf. Guess what? I found them.

I repackaged the mango slices, dropping each of them in its own individual wallet-size plastic bag. The strategy worked for a while. I felt guilty about unzipping fifteen bags to have fifteen portions a day. But it became too time-consuming to prepare, not to mention plastic-bag-consuming.

Sometimes, before padding out to the kitchen, I'd look at the digitally aged picture of Old A.J. Should I do this to him? Well, I think he'd forgive me. I've found Old A.J. is better for motivating me to take action—go to the gym, hop on the treadmill, have a cucumber—than he is at stopping my vices.

The other day, though, I had a breakthrough. I listened to a segment on the great science show *Radiolab* about bad habits. It featured an interview with Thomas Schelling—the Nobel Prize–winning economist who came up with now-self-vs.-future-self concept of egonomics.

He talked about an antismoking strategy that sounded intriguing. It was worth a shot, I figured.

When Julie got home, I asked her a favor.

"If I have another dried mango this month, I want you to donate a thousand dollars of my money to the American Nazi Party."

"The Nazi Party? Why not Oxfam?"

"That's not enough of a disincentive. I want something that will make me sick to my stomach."

"Ah, right," said Julie.

She quickly got into the spirit. She filled out a check to the Nazi Party, signed it, and wrote "Courtesy of A.J. Jacobs" in the memo space. She waved it in front of me. "Don't eat any of those dried mangoes—as delicious they may be."

This is what's known as an "Odysseus Contract." In *The Odyssey*, our crafty hero demanded that his sailors tie him to the mast so that he wouldn't take a dive off the starboard side when he heard the alluring singing of the Sirens. You shouldn't trust your future self. Prepare for his weaknesses.

Thank God for Odysseus. Because let me tell you: This strategy is one of the most effective I've ever encountered. I haven't eaten a dried mango in two weeks.

I still open the cabinet, and see those slices, and get a few drops of Pavlovian saliva. But there's no way I'm going to put one in my mouth. It's like a switch has been flipped. I can't even conceive of eating one. The repercussions are too horrible. I'm not going to pay for a bunch of new swastika flags and jackboot laces.

It's as if I were dating a woman and discovered she was my long-lost sister. The thought of kissing her repulses.

It's been two weeks, and I haven't eaten a single slice. I'm a hero.

The no-sugar diet is ridiculously hard to sustain, and sustain it I won't. But just two weeks of sugar fasting improved how I felt. I had more energy, fewer aches and pains, and better workouts. As always, the placebo effect shouldn't be discounted. But I've become more antisugar as a result of this mini-experiment.

I'm a weak man, so after the two weeks were over, I started using a sugar substitute called stevia. Sugar haters say it's a crutch, and may raise insulin resistance. But most believe that, as far as sugar substitutes go, stevia is the healthiest. You can buy stevia in leaf form, or as little packets of powder. It has a vanilla taste, so I'm enjoying some vanilla-infused steel-cut oatmeal, and broccoli puree that tastes a bit like ice cream.

In my final act of defiance against King Sugar, I decide to try to cut sweet talk from my language as well. I shouldn't glorify sugar's taste by calling Julie by my usual pet name, "sweetie." Calling her "savory" didn't sound so romantic, so I settled on "pumpkin," even though it's kind of starchy. She approved.

Checkup: Month 16

Weight: 157 (dropped to 154 when eating raw food)

Miles walked while writing this book: 1012 (broke the grand mark)

Meals this month with bok choy: 12

Meals with bok choy 1968–2009: 0

Most steps in a single day: 21,340 (walking to Tribeca, plus a
lot of housecleaning)

This month, I joined my mom and dad for their respective workouts. Research shows that spending time with the family is healthy, assuming you don't despise your family, which I don't, thankfully.

My mom took me to her Pilates studio, with its collection of machines made of leather, wood, and cables. They look as if they were jointly designed by Eric Roberts in *Star 80* and Tomás de Torquemada. They have vaguely threatening names like "The Reformer."

The workout itself wasn't too scary, though. "We get to run while lying down," my mom told me. I had to agree that's a pretty good deal.

My dad's workout was more traditional: Treadmill trotting and strength training at a gym near his midtown office.

I never imagined I'd be working out with my parents. Mostly because, growing up, my parents weren't exercise enthusiasts. They emphasized intellect. My dad spent his free time reading the *Encyclopedia Britannica* and writing law books. (He holds the record for the most footnotes in a law review article: 4,824.)

Athletics just weren't high on the agenda. It's only now, as they've gotten older, that they've started to exercise in earnest.

My childhood biases run deep, though. I often feel guilty that I'm spending so much time on my body. Shouldn't I be busy improving my brain instead of my delts?

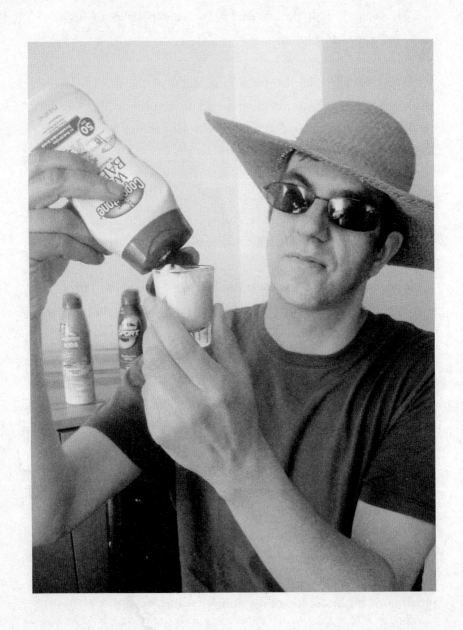

Chapter 17

The Skin

The Quest to Erase Blemishes

I'VE BEEN RESEARCHING THE VARIOUS OINTMENTS, chemicals, and sprays that humans apply to their faces in their quest for healthy skin. Or healthy-looking skin, in any case.

And it's an astonishing list, ranging from the delicious to the unimaginably repulsive.

In the appetizing category: yogurt, lemon, walnut oil, honey, almonds, avocados, mint, and pumpkin. The foreheads in Beverly Hills are better fed than the average laborer in an equatorial nation.

On the other hand, people also pay to have an alarming assortment of bodily fluids applied to their face. A New York spa will spread bird excrement on your pores for two hundred dollars. Another spa will shine your skin with spermine, an antioxidant originally found in sperm that has now been manufactured in Norway. Snail secretion facials are also available. Seems we haven't come so far from Elizabethan times, when there was a fad for puppy urine skin cleanser.

Skin treatments are not a new trend. In the Old Testament book of Esther, the evil king needs a new queen, so he holds an *American Idol*–style contest. Every night, he sleeps with a different woman. But not before the contestant has undergone beauty treatments that last *an entire year*. Six months with oil of myrrh, and six months with spices. Which makes a half hour in front of the mirror before a first date seem reasonable.

In my forty-two years, I'd never put anything delicious or disgusting on my face, apart from suntan lotion and face paint during camp color war. Why should I? I figured my skin can take care of itself. Don't micromanage.

But recently I got paranoid that I'm the last man in modern times with no skin-care regimen at all. I was in the Penn Station bathroom before heading off to Philadelphia, when I overheard two guys talking. Leather jackets, Harley tattoos, belt-obscuring guts. They were either bikers or overzealous undercover cops.

"The sun is fucking killing me. I'm moisturizing like crazy. I'm using every fucking thing. I'm using fucking aloe. The whole thing."

The other shook his head in sympathetic exasperation.

As part of the project, I have to take care of my skin. Skin cancer is the most common form of cancer in the world. There are two million cases a year in the United States alone, according to the American Cancer Society. And on a more superficial level, as my Penn Station friends can tell you, your skin broadcasts your age. This month is the month of skin.

Smoothing Things Over

But what skin products to apply? Skin care is estimated to be a $43 billion industry, and the quackery level is astoundingly high. Doctor and journalist Ben Goldacre gives a thorough lashing to the skin cream industry in his book *Bad Science*. They throw in scientific-sounding ingredients like "specially treated salmon roe DNA." If your skin actually did absorb salmon DNA, Goldacre points out, you might grow scales, which would appeal to a niche group.

The skin-care choices are dizzying (see Appendix). But Goldacre writes that unless you have a skin problem, one moisturizer is almost as good as any other. For now, I'm using my wife's Aveeno lotion.

Wrinkles are a different story. Of all the dozens of wrinkle-preventing options, just a few actually work. The most established: tretinoin, known more widely as Retin-A. This acid helps the skin retain collagen, the elastic material. It might even have health benefits in addition to the cosmetic ones. According to the *New York Times*, it's been used to treat precancerous skin cells. Studies show that after two years of use, abnormal cells returned to normal.

At my request, my dermatologist prescribed me a tube of Retin-A. It's absurdly expensive—eighty dollars for two ounces. I decided to submit a claim just to give the insurance guy a good belly laugh.

I started spreading the thick, white lotion around my eyes and forehead. A week. Nothing. Two weeks. Nothing. Third week . . . something? The fourth week, definitely something.

The deep cracks around my eyes remained, but the little crevices filled out, like an inflating balloon.

It wasn't a placebo effect: I asked Julie.

"You look younger," she tells me. "It's weird."

"You can borrow it if you want."

"Why?" Julie says. "Do you think I need it?"

Huh. This is one of those Joe Pesci–style "do you think I'm a clown?" questions. There's no winning. You end up backpedaling and being shot in the foot with a Glock 19, if only metaphorically.

Julie did borrow my tube, and it backfired on her. Her skin got all red and puffy. "You'll have to deal with wrinkled old me," she said as she gave me back the tube.

I went back to dabbing it on each night. I watched the tiny dents in my face erode like a handprint in the rising tide. I spent an embarrassing amount of time in the mirror studying the skin around my eyes. I never thought of myself as being concerned about mini-wrinkles. Who cares? They add character, right?

And yet, it's an astonishing feeling to watch such a clear cause and effect. Apply cream, wrinkles vanish. It's like Photoshop, but in real life.

Then I started studying the rest of my face. What else can I fix? What about that chin? It sort of flows smoothly into the throat, creating a combined chin/throat: a choat.

Or maybe my slightly asymmetrical nose? Maybe I should get that fixed.

I snapped out of it after a couple of minutes. I remind myself that vanity is more addictive than most Schedule IV drugs.

I can see how this quest for physical perfection might slide into insanity. How a reality-show star can have forty-three plastic surgeries in a month and how author Alex Kuczynski can sustain a whole book on beauty junkies.

Plus Retin-A has other downsides. It makes skin more likely to get sunburned as it allows in more UV light. And God knows what other unforeseen side effects will bubble up over the years. Not to mention that it's a money vacuum.

So on a random Wednesday, I put the Retin-A in the back of

my closet. Though maybe I'll start up again for the book tour. You know, for business purposes.

The Bronze Age

When I was a kid, sunscreen rarely touched my body. I loved a good tan, which I somehow thought made me look less scrawny. As a result, my skin is a canvas of craters and crow's-feet and splotches.

I was kindly reminded of this on a recent vacation. We met a fellow tourist who remarked that Julie and I looked young. We smiled. Until her husband, a dermatologist, replied:

"No, they don't. I can see a lot of skin damage. A huge amount."

He guessed, correctly, that we were in our forties. Julie still hasn't forgiven him. "Unless you work at a carnival, keep your age guesses to yourself," she said.

But he's right about our skin damage.

And for this, I've decided to blame Coco Chanel. In researching suntans, I found out the French designer is considered the godmother of modern bronzing. For centuries, middle-class white people avoided tans for fear of looking like they worked in the field like a common peasant. But in 1923, Coco Chanel vacationed in the Mediterranean on the yacht of an aristocrat friend, and was spotted on board with a deep tan. Caramel-colored skin soon became the rage, the sign that you could afford a sun-drenched holiday.

After learning this story, I added Coco Chanel to my list of the top-five health villains. Think of how many cases of fatal skin cancer this woman is responsible for. Thousands? Millions? Maybe that's too harsh. Maybe I shouldn't be angry at this delightfully chic lady, the creator of plumed hats and Marilyn Monroe's nighttime wear ("five drops of Chanel No. 5"). Maybe we shouldn't fault her and her alone. Maybe. But in my defense, Coco Chanel had some other rather serious flaws. She had a notorious years-long affair with a Nazi spy during the occupation, and was later charged by the French government as a collaborator. (She escaped trial only thanks to intervention by her friends in the British royal family.) Which makes her life especially ironic—she was involved with two opposed evils: white supremacy and tanning.

Coco Chanel needed more sunscreen. A lot more. As do most of us. When Americans put on sunscreen, we underapply the stuff, using about a quarter to half of the correct amount, say dermatologists.

The American Academy of Dermatology suggests a shot-glass-ful of sunscreen every two to four hours. You should apply it regardless of the weather—whether it's cloudy (80 percent of UV rays penetrate clouds) or winter (especially with snow, which reflects sunlight).

So, on a Saturday morning, before walking our kids to a friend's birthday party, I squeezed my Coppertone Sport Broad Spectrum UVA/UVB sunscreen (plus antioxidant defense) until it filled a shot glass, and then dipped my finger in and started slathering it on my body.

A shot glass is about 1 to 1.5 ounces. It's hard to comprehend just how much sunscreen this is unless you try it yourself. Go ahead, I'll wait. Still waiting. You see? You're probably exhausted from squeezing the sunscreen tube, right?

With my shot glass, I had enough sunscreen to coat my body four times. I glistened like a Mr. Universe contestant, only without the distracting abs.

"I've run out of body parts," Julie said, when she tried to do it. "And I think I got it in my mouth. The dermatologists have to be getting kickbacks from the sunscreen companies."

Applying it every two hours, Julie and I emptied an entire eight-ounce bottle in a single day. We finished more than half of another bottle for the boys.

When I tell my aunt Marti, she's appalled. She thinks sunscreen is filled with toxins. I'm avoiding scented sunscreens, which might have phthalates, but otherwise, I'm ignoring the risk. Sorry, Marti, again.

Some vitamin-D advocates are also skeptical of sunscreen. For the last few months, D has been the trendiest of all vitamins, the Lady Gaga of supplements (or whichever pop star the bar mitzvah DJs are playing ad nauseam these days). Its fans—such as Dr. Sarfraz Zaidi, a professor of medicine at UCLA—say vitamin-D deficiency is linked to cancer, heart disease, diabetes, kidney disease, chronic fatigue, asthma, dental problems, and depression, among many, many other ills.

Not counting supplements, we get vitamin D from foods such as salmon and egg yolks, and sun exposure, which let us synthesize it ourselves. The D fans say that we use too much sunscreen and suppress our levels.

The quarrel between dermatologists and vitamin-D advocates is an example of a problem infecting all medicine: the specialty bias. Most experts see the world through the prism of their specialty.

Based on my advisory board's counsel, I'm taking a middle path: exposing one sunscreen-free limb every other day for fifteen minutes. I vary the limb, to reduce the chances of overexposure to any particular part.

The Mole

Among my skin's many imperfections: I have a mole on the side of my nose.

Had I been alive 250 years ago in France, this would have been quite a boon. I read in the encyclopedia that back in the days of Louis XV, there was a vogue for moles. Black patches of gummed taffeta were popular with chic women and men who wanted to emphasize the beauty and whiteness of their skin. The smart set had plenty of patch designs to choose from. For the understated, there were the simple spots. But the truly fashionable had patches in the shapes of stars, crescents, elaborate animals, insects, or figures. Placement was also important, seeing as these patches had their own language: A patch at the corner of the eye symbolized passion, while one at the middle of the forehead indicated dignity. Women carried their patch boxes with them, in case they wanted to slap on a fresh one during the royal ball.

My mole, sadly, isn't in the shape of a giraffe or spider. Just a regular old spot, about the size and color of a chocolate chip. And unfortunately, instead of inspiring coquettish smiles and fluttering eyelids from ladies of the court, it inspires lingering stares that lie on the border between curious and dismayed.

After a visit to the dermatologist—not the insulting one, a kindly friend of the family named Dr. Eileen Lambroza—I decide to have it removed—as well as the mole on my back, which is actually more worrisome to her, since it's asymmetrical.

A mole—the medical term is "nevus"—is an abnormal clump of skin cells that produce the brownish-black pigment melanin. Caucasian adults each have an average of thirty moles on their bodies. And it's not a small health problem: More than a million Americans are diagnosed with skin cancer every year. And worldwide, at least fifty thousand die each year of skin cancer that came from moles, according to the World Health Organization.

A few days later, I'm in the office of a plastic surgeon, an Orthodox Jewish man. He's wearing those glasses with miniature telescopes protruding from the lenses. He studies my mole, before announcing his analysis.

"That thing is the size of Providence!"

Well, at least he chose a midsize city without much suburban sprawl.

The surgery took all of twenty minutes. I couldn't see what was happening, but I felt a needle prick, heard some emery-board-like scratching, smelled burning skin, and felt thread tugging at my nostril.

The doctor was nice and apparently at the top of his field. He was also talkative. I knew from my research on multitasking that chatting can interfere with performance. So I answered his questions in monosyllables. No, I didn't speak Polish. Not much happening at work. I felt guilty being terse.

When I got home, Julie was at her desk paying some bills. She looked up. For a few seconds, she peered at me like she was trying to solve a four-dimensional topology problem.

"You got your mole taken off?"

I nodded.

"You didn't tell me? No warning? No debate?"

I shrugged.

"It's such a part of you. You've had it forty-two years."

I could see tears welling up. Actual tears. I didn't expect this much emotion over a hunk of melanin. I got nervous.

"So I should have kept it?"

"No, I'm happy about it. Overwhelmingly happy. I never wanted to say what I thought about it before . . ."

They were tears of relief and surprise, not sadness. Interesting. We've been married more than a decade, but Julie's never brought up my mole, for fear of hurting my feelings. What other secret opinions does she have that she's too polite to say?

A week later, Dr. Lambroza called with the results of the biopsy. The nose mole was fine. But the one on my back, well . . .

"It was atypical."

Huh. That doesn't sound good. Atypical is fine when it comes to movie tastes, but medically, I want to be as dull, boring and typical as possible.

"It didn't qualify as cancerous. There weren't enough atypical features to diagnose it as a melanoma. But it was still atypical. It's a good thing you're writing this book and you had a dermatology appointment," she says.

If I hadn't caught it, it would probably have turned into cancer in a few years.

There it is, another little wake-up call about mortality. A tiny wake-up call. Not a noble or impressive one. Nothing that would get me a get me a lot of sympathy at the corner bar, but a wake-up call nonetheless. My body is filled with imperfections, and one of them will get me.

Checkup: Month 17

Weight: 161 (creeping back up)

"I am grateful for" e-mails exchanged with mother: 27

Personal record for most superfoods eaten in one meal: 11
    (salad with black currants, red peppers, wheat germ, cooked
    shiitake mushrooms blueberries, avocados, pomegranite
    seeds, lentils, mango, flaxseed oil, almonds)

Trips to the gym this month: 11

Yes, my gym attendance is shameful. My running schedule isn't much better—three times a week instead of everyday at my peak. I need motivation. I've realized 80 percent of this year is about motivation. Most health advice can be summed up in five words: *Eat less, move more, relax.* The question is: How do you do that? That is my struggle.

How do you gag the voice in your head that says, "You don't have to go to the gym today. There's always out tomorrow. C'mon, my friend, it's just one plate of curly fries. Yes, just for you!" (My inner voice reminds me of a particularly aggressive rug salesman at a Turkish bazaar.)

Motivation will be next month's theme.

My friend Charles Duhigg—a reporter for the *New York Times*—is working on a book about developing good habits. He tells me that one important element is rewarding yourself. So after every workout, I've been rewarding myself with ten minutes of the sleazy, lowbrow, but highly entertaining gossip site TMZ.com. It's helpful, as is my photo of Old A.J. But I need more.

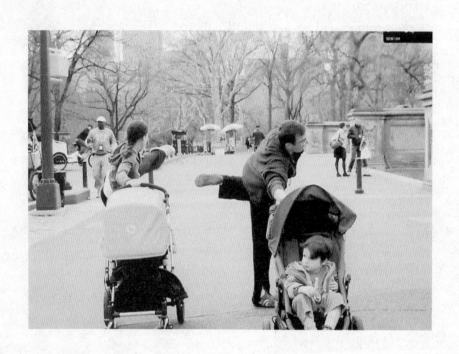

Chapter 18

The Heart, Revisited

The Quest for the Perfect Workout

THE SOLUTION TO MY LACKLUSTER workout schedule, I decide, is to mix things up. Try new activities. Feed my short attention span a bit of aerobic variety. Fortunately, the number of workout options is stunning. It reminds me of my year of living biblically, with the hundreds of different denominations, each with fervent believers devoted to their leader.

So I try a bunch. I try a sadistic ballet-yoga-aerobics cocktail called Physique 57, favored by Kelly Ripa. I try yoga. Then I try AntiGravity yoga, where you move through your poses in your own orange, cocoonlike hammock that hangs from the ceiling.

I take a class for new moms (and dads) called "Strollercise," where I push Zane's Maclaren stroller while jogging and jumping and stretching and getting stared at in Central Park. I try CrossFit training, a high-intensity workout in a low-tech gym filled with bar-bells and medicine balls. Working out to exhaustion is encouraged. CrossFit's mascot is named Pukey.

One trainer gives me the Roman Legionnaire's Workout, which involves smashing logs in Central Park with a huge metal mallet. Typical feedback from passersby on the walk home: "Hey, are you Thor?"

And today, I'm trying another: pole dancing. As I mentioned early on, it's the most popular class at my gym, so I figured I should check it out.

Before I begin, let's get something straight: Pole dancing has nothing to do with stripping. Aside from the technicality that 95 percent of it takes place at strip clubs.

At least this is the position of pole-dancing evangelists. Pole dancing is an art form, like a vertical ballet. Or a sport, like gymnastics, only with more pelvic gyrations. But it's not sleazy.

Their line of argument is a tad whitewashed, for sure. But after my pole-dancing session, I can say that the gist is true: Hanging and twirling on a pole will get your ventricles and atria pumping.

When I arrive, thanks to years of training as a sharp-eyed journalist, I observe that I'm the only man. Fifty women and me. This ratio turns out to be common in almost all my classes, not just those involving G-strings and erotic dance. When it comes to fitness, Americans like to reinforce stereotypes: Women prefer community. Men are rugged individualists.

The instructor, a Latina with close-cropped hair, takes us through a series of warm-up stretches and hip thrusts. Here's where I expend a lot of energy trying not to act or feel creepy. I'm here as a professional, after all. This goal is made much more difficult by several factors. For instance, the instructor repeatedly yells phrases such as "really spread your legs!" Also the outfits don't help. I try not to stare, but trying to avoid cleavage here is like trying to avoid old white guys on the Senate floor. It's omnipresent.

After fifteen minutes of warm-up to, what else, Lady Gaga, we choose a pole. I'm alarmed to find out that we aren't given our own individual pole. You share with three other dancers. I'm assigned to a pole in the corner with a trio of women, each one wearing a different-colored pair of high heels (red, black, and white).

Anna (red) is up first. She's part Asian and part Swedish. Her T-shirt reads I HAVE A HEART-ON FOR PEACE.

She grabs the pole and does the back hook, the chair, the jump and slide, the fireman's turn. She wraps her legs around the pole, she slides upside down, arches her back.

Then she grabs a towel and wipes down the pole. Dr. Tierno would be proud.

My turn. I try to remember the tips from our instructor: "Keep your hips away from the pole when you're climbing, because otherwise you just look desperate." And "If you don't have heels, remember to point your toes."

I did my best, but as you might expect, my performance resembled a fourth-grade asthmatic trying to climb the rope in gym class.

"I'm impressed that you're trying," says Anna. I recognize the tone: It's what I use when Lucas is trying to read a five-letter word.

"I think I got pole burn," I say. I point to my red calf. Anna gives me a knowing nod.

"Look at this." Anna points to her own legs, which are dotted with brown bruises. "You get used to it. I don't even feel it anymore."

Turns out Anna is a ringer. She's president of the U.S. Pole Dance Federation and is organizing next month's national championships. When she finds out I work at *Esquire*, she tells me that she'd love it if the magazine would cover the event. She writes down her phone number on a scrap of paper.

When I get home, I show Julie that I have gotten the digits of pole dancing's most powerful official. "So proud of you!" she says.

The Goal

Friends keep trying to recruit me to their own fitness classes. "Oh, you will *love* Zumba." Or hula hooping. Or faith-based aerobics, whatever that is.

Julie got me to attend a class at her gym. The teacher spent the class sitting comfortably in her chair at the front of the room and yelling at us to lift our glutes. I found it offensive. If you're going to shout about glute-lifting, at least lift a glute or two yourself, right? The instructor's obesity added to my skepticism.

The variety strategy is backfiring. It's getting numbing instead of inspiring. It almost always boils down to moving your arms and legs in a room with mirrors.

I need another way to motivate myself to exercise. Maybe I need a goal. All my fitness books talk about goals. You need a goal, and preferably a publicly and loudly stated one, one whose failure results in high levels of humiliation. But what goal?

"Why don't you do a triathlon?" Julie asks one night as we scrub our BPA-free dishes.

"I don't know," I say. "It doesn't seem so healthy."

At the start of my project, I considered a triathlon, but dismissed it. I'd even watched a few YouTube videos on triathlons, including one that purported to be a motivational video. It featured stumbling runners collapsing on the road and convulsing. There was a woman on a stretcher. With an IV in her arm. That kind of motivation does not work on me. When I watch *Saw III*, I don't say to myself, "Hey, I really want to be chained up in a sociopath's basement." Same idea.

Though triathlons have an aura of fitness about them, I'm not sure they're maximally healthy. Between 2006 and 2008, fourteen people died while doing triathlons, either from heart attacks or drowning. Triathletes abuse their joints. Extreme endurance sports, according to some studies, lower life spans. Or maybe these are just studies designed by lazy people to reinforce their choices.

But Julie pressed on.

"You don't have to do the ones that make you vomit blood. You could do a smaller one."

Maybe she had a point. A smaller race would still get me training. And also, I could tell my friends that, yes, I finished a triathlon, which is sort of the fitness equivalent of doing the haftorah at your bar mitzvah. It'd make a man of me.

When I looked online, I found hundreds of triathlons of varying lengths. Since their origins in 1902 in France, "tris," as those in the know call them, have grown into a $500-million-per-year industry worldwide. (Incidentally, that first triathlon featured canoeing instead of swimming, which sounds much drier and more pleasant.)

Yes, there's the famed Ironman triathlon—five-2.4 mile swim, 112-mile bike ride, twenty-six-mile run. But then there are also ones barely more strenuous than a jog around the block.

Julie's right. I can do one. But which one? I was drawn to the triathlon that was conducted entirely indoors—treadmill, stationary bike, and lap pool. That seemed comfortable. But sadly, as we know, indoor exercise isn't as healthy as outdoor exercise. I'd have to expose myself to the elements.

I found a race in Staten Island on May 5, just a couple of months away. It was eminently conquerable—twelve-mile bike ride, three-mile run, and quarter-mile swim in open water. It's an oxymoronic challenge: a moderate extreme sport. My medical advisers were always yapping on about "everything in moderation." So here it was, the healthiest triathlon possible.

The next day, I announced to Julie, my friends, and my sons: "I'm doing a triathlon."

I call Julie's friend Anna, a remarkable athlete and veteran of several triathlons. I tell her I'm joining her ranks and ask her for advice.

"I did a triathlon in early May," she says. "The water is freezing. It's horrible. I cried."

That doesn't sound moderate.

Fast and Furious

I've been reading *Aesop's Fables* to the boys. And I've developed a soft spot for the much maligned hare in the story of the tortoise and the hare.

(I'm also, by the way, a fan of the fox who rationalized that the out-of-reach grapes were sour. That was some good reframing, Fox).

But back to the hare. The long-eared fellow might have been onto something—and not just because naps are healthy.

The hare's method has advantages, especially when training for a triathlon.

The hare was essentially doing what's now known as High-Intensity Interval Training (HIIT). Instead of jogging at 60 percent of your ability for forty-five minutes, you go at 100 percent for a mere thirty seconds. Then you stop and rest for a minute. Then sprint again. Then repeat eight times. Total time: twelve minutes. Or less, if you scale back on the rest periods.

It's an astounding time-saver. And growing evidence shows it might be just as effective as long, moderate exercise. Not just for elite athletes, but for everyone, including the obese.

The catch is, it hurts. "There's no free lunch," Martin Gibala of McMasters University, one of the HIIT experts told me. It's akin to the Band-Aid Removal Preference Dilemma: Would you rather rip it off quickly (intense pain, but over in a flash)? Or pull it off slowly (wee bit of pain, but drags on much longer).

HIIT is the aerobic cousin of the super-slow weights workout I did with Adam Zickerman. But it has more studies to back up its big claims.

To take one of the most famous: In a 1996 study by University of Tokyo professor Mikito Tabata, athletes spent twenty seconds huffing as hard as possible on a specially designed stationary bike, followed by ten-second rest. They did this for a total of four minutes, four times a week. At month's end, they showed amazing gains in their metabolism—more than those athletes who pedaled at a moderate pace for forty-five minutes per session (what's known as steady-state exercise, with a whiff of condescension).

The benefits are many: raised endurance, lower blood sugar, improved lung capacity, and weight loss. HIIT seems to alter the metabolism and muscle structure, so you burn more calories throughout the day.

Tony gave me a HIIT session today. We used a stationary bicycle, since running full-speed can be hard on the joints.

We cranked up the bike all the way.

"Now go as fast as you can!"

Tony once told me that in some L.A. gyms, people keep their faces deadpan like Buster Keaton. They don't want to cause wrinkles.

But today, I needed to grimace. And grunt. And shut my eyes and rock my head back and forth like Stevie Wonder.

I'm doing HIIT only once a week. First, because there need to be more long-term studies—such as whether it prevents heart disease as well as normal exercise. And second, because it makes me nauseated.

Checkup: Month 18

Weight: 159

Push-ups till exhaustion: 100 (!)

Percentage of fruits and vegetables organic: 60

Days I activated Freedom software (prevents Internet access,
   thus lowering stress and improving concentration): 19

Days I rebooted my computer in order to short-circuit
   Freedom software: 15

My big accomplishment this month is that I set up an interview
with Jack LaLanne. He's ninety-six and still going. He's not tugging
seventy boats behind him as he swims across Long Beach Harbor,
as he did on his seventieth birthday. But he's still going.

The date has taken a while to set up. He's a busy man. When I
first approached him, I got this e-mail from his assistant. "Jack has
been in New Jersey all week, shooting a new juicer infomercial.
We will get back to you next week. Healthfully, Claire." As far as
excuses go, a juicer commercial is probably the favorite I've ever
received.

But now it's all come together, and I've bought a plane ticket to
see him at his home in Morro Bay, California. His house has two
gyms and a swimming pool that he still uses every day.

I love researching LaLanne. I knew he was early on the fitness
train, but I didn't know what a rebel he was. "People thought I was
a charlatan and a nut," he said. "The doctors were against me. They
said working out with weights would give people heart attacks and
they'd lose their sex drive."

He started out as a junk-food addict, but had his Road-to-
Damascus moment when he was fifteen and attended a health
lecture. His diet from then on consisted of raw fruits, vegetables,

fish, oatmeal, and egg whites—come to think of it, pretty much my diet. Our lifestyles are remarkably similar. Except he avoids coffee. Also, he used to drink a daily quart of blood. Oh, and he could tow seventy boats while swimming across the harbor on his seventieth birthday.

His quotes are both hilarious and inspiring: "Fifteen minutes to warm up? Does a lion warm up when he's hungry? 'Uh-oh, here comes an antelope. Better warm up.' No! He just goes out there and eats the sucker." I printed that out and put it on my wall next to the passage from Carl Sagan.

Along with healthy eating and lots of exercise, the third pillar of Jack's lifestyle is sleep. He goes to bed between 9 and 10 p.m. (though he is nearly a hundred years old, so I guess that's not exactly a shocker). But it's good motivation. I need to work on my nighttime health.

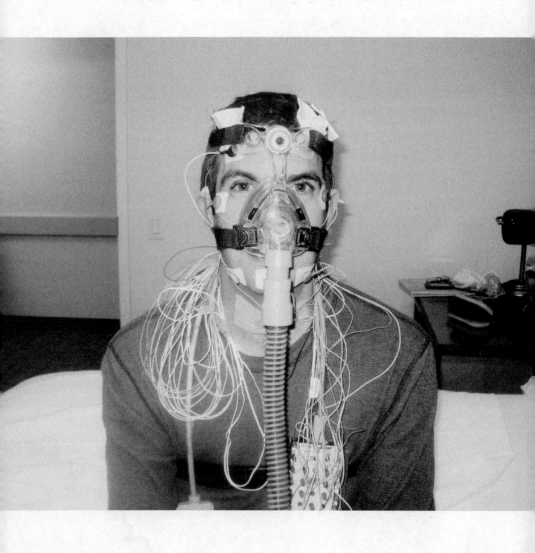

Chapter 19

The Inside of the Eyelid

The Quest for the Perfect Night's Sleep

I ENVY DOLPHINS. Not so much for their grace or power, but because of the way they sleep. Dolphins sleep one half brain at a time. When the right side of their brain is asleep, the left side is awake. And vice versa. They developed this skill because they need to be conscious enough to return to the surface every few minutes for a gulp of air.

Why couldn't evolution have come up with this system for us? It's so frustrating. Think of all we could do while half asleep. All the bills I could pay, the *Esquire* meetings I could sit, through, the children's birthday parties I could attend.

Instead, we're stuck with this absurd, eyes-shut, openmouthed, dead-to-the-world system. I hate sleep. I spend one-third of my life drooling on my pillow.

Julie, on the other hand, is a huge fan. Sleeping is her favorite hobby. She talks about a good night's sleep in rapturous tones, like a jazz lover talking about a Miles Davis solo at the Blue Note. She could sleep for fourteen hours a day.

She's so fixated, she blames any health problem our family confronts on lack of sleep. Cold, flu, infection, sore elbow—you just need more sleep, she'll say.

Sadly for me, she's not far off. More and more studies show undersleeping's deadly sway. It contributes to heart disease and hypertension. It hobbles our immune system. In the United States, one hundred thousand sleep-related car crashes occur every year. It impairs our cognitive function, effectively lowering our IQ and our ability to pay attention. It costs the U.S. economy an estimated $63 billion a year.

I sleep about six hours a night, and spend a lot of my day exhausted, as if there's a twenty-pound weight pressing down on the top of my head.

Here's how tired I am: Several times in the last few weeks, I fell asleep while reading books to my sons. I'm proud to say that these naps didn't stop me from finishing the book. It's just that the plots took on a more Dadaist tone.

I'm not sure what the phrase "three-alarm cabinet" means, but when I heard myself utter it while reading a *Corduroy* the bear story, I knew I'd dozed off. I jolted myself awake. Then fell asleep again.

Maybe I'd be more enamored of sleep if I were good at it. I just don't have Julie's talent for it. I snore, I go to sleep too late, and I can't fall asleep when I'm finally in bed. These are the dragons I have to slay.

Noisy Night at Home

Julie has always told me that I snore at leaf-blower levels. Plus I thrash around like I'm having a seizure. And I tend to illegally occupy her mattress territory, even if we're at a hotel with one of the fourteen-foot-wide dictator-size beds.

This has resulted in our marriage's shameful secret, which I'll reveal here. I hope you won't judge: We don't sleep together often. I'm not talking having sex together. I'm talking going through REM cycles in the same room.

About five years ago, she told me she'd had enough. Whenever possible, I should find another place to sleep. Ever since, I've been spending most nights in the home office.

A couple of months ago, the *New York Times* ran an article about separated-at-night couples. We're part of a trend. A survey by the National Association of Home Builders says 60 percent of custom houses will have dual master bedrooms by 2015.

It's still a bit taboo, though. Too Victorian for modern tastes. Me, I'm happy to come out of my separate closet. Julie was more reluctant, but has fessed up to it in recent years. We both think it has advantages. She doesn't have to listen to my snoring, and I can go to bed whenever I want without worrying about disturbing her.

So I'm not sure whether we'll ever return to the same sleeping bed. But regardless, I need to fix the original cause of the nocturnal separation: the snoring.

Snoring is linked to a host of horrible problems: fatigue, of course, but also heart disease, depression, and car accidents. Snoring occurs when your airways are obstructed. It could be the tongue falling back into the throat, or lack of air through nasal passageways, or fatty tissues in the throat—any number of things.

Snoring could also be a symptom of sleep apnea, a more serious condition in which the air passages are blocked and the sleeper stops breathing altogether for several seconds, if not minutes.

I visit Dr. Steven Park, antisnoring crusader and author of *Sleep, Interrupted* in his midtown office. He wants to take a look at my airways. I wince as he pokes a probe up my nose and down my throat.

He sits on a stool and breaks the news to me. My nose has a deviated septum, says Dr. Park. Very deviated, zigzagging this way and that like San Francisco's Lombard Street. "It's a really complicated curved septum," he says. "There's complex geometry." He also calls me a mouth breather, which I try to remind myself is a diagnosis, not an insult.

"I can tell you right now, there's no simple fix," Dr. Park told me. "For the average snorer, it's a journey."

Over the course of the next two weeks, I try no fewer than twenty remedies. A handful of highlights include:

The Tennis Ball Cure

Snoring is most severe when you sleep on your back. The tongue collapses down toward your throat and blocks the air. It's better to sleep on your side. One classic remedy is to sew a tennis ball into the back of your pajamas. I'm not much with needlework, but I do know how to use duct tape, so I taped a Wilson U.S. Open ball to my T-shirt.

The problem is, I slept on my back despite the ball. Apparently, if I were a damsel in that fairy tale with the pea and the mattress, I'd never be allowed to marry the prince. I'm too comfortable in uncomfortable positions.

The Pillow

I order Brookstone's antisnoring memory foam neck Pillow for seventy dollars. It keeps my head elevated and my chin out, which helps the airways stay open. It's like sleeping on a giant gummi bear.

The neck pillow worked a bit. I've been tape-recording myself every night, and listening back in the morning. (Which is kind of creepy. I feel like I'm invading my own privacy.) But Julie's not lying. I am loud. The good news: I noted about a 10 percent drop in snoring. Progress!

Tongue Exercises

I start a regimen of antisnoring exercises meant to firm up the tongue and throat muscles (though the scientific evidence on them seems flimsy). At night I do ten minutes in front of my computer: Pucker-hold-smile-hold, then flick your tongue from corner to corner. Julie spots my tongue-flicking. "What kind of websites are you looking at?" she wants to know.

The Didgeridoo

There are studies by actual accredited scientists, including one published in the *British Medical Journal*, that say that playing this Australian aboriginal instrument strengthens the throat muscles and helps cure snoring.

The didgeridoo, I learn from the instruction manual, is the world's oldest wind instrument, made when termites hollow out a eucalyptus branch. My didge, brown with red stripes, arrives in a skinny cardboard box.

It takes me a day to figure out how to position my lips to get the low, droning foghornlike sound. When I do, my kids think it's hilarious, as it's vaguely flatulent. I also played a deep version of "Happy Birthday" for one of my friends, which she pretended to appreciate.

Is the didgeridoo helping? Hard to say, but my friend Shannon pointed out that it keeps my neighbors up, preventing *them* from snoring. So that's something.

Breathe Right Strip

This is the tape that you strap over your nose to widen the nostrils. I try it that night. "You look angry," says Julie, pointing to my flared nostrils. But I love the rush of air I get from the strips. It gives me such a boost of energy, I'm worried I won't be able to fall asleep. But I do. I listen to my digital tape recorder. There's wheezing, but much less outright snorting. More progress!

The Sleep Clinic

If I want to stop snoring altogether, I've got to take more serious measures. Dr. Park suggests I make a visit to New York's renowned Sleep Disorders Institute for an overnight study.

I show up, and a technician leads me to a room with bare, white walls and a bed. The most colorful things in my sleep chamber are the wires that a technician spends forty-five minutes taping to my head, chest, and legs. The wires are yellow, green, red, purple, and orange, making me look like a convicted murderer at a festive execution. I also have tubes up my nose and in front of my mouth.

The doctors monitor everything: heart rate, oxygen, brain activity, and nasal exhalations. I toss and turn for two hours before I finally fall asleep, then wake up feeling grimy and do a walk-of-shame-like trip back to my apartment. Dr. Park calls a couple of days later.

I woke up a few times.

"How many?" I ask.

"A hundred eighty-five," Dr. Park says.

I don't know how to respond. That's 180 more than what I would have guessed.

Dr. Park's voice remains calm. Actually, he says, it's not too bad. Patients with severe sleep apnea wake hundreds of times. But I do have a "mild case" of sleep apnea.

At one point, I stopped breathing for forty-two seconds, sending my oxygen level down. Which is worrisome, to say the least. Sleep apnea is a big problem, a contributor to heart disease, fatigue, and brain damage.

The best cure for sleep apnea is something called a CPAP machine (short for Continuous Positive Airway Pressure). You put a mask on your face attached to a hose that shoots air down your nose and mouth to keep the airways open.

I return to the institute for another night to get fitted. My technician this time, Alison—a petite but tough former paramedic—straps the mask on my nose and turns on the air hose. I feel like a golden retriever with my head stuck out of a car window.

I'm supposed to sleep like this?

"You'll get used to it," she assures me, then turns out the light.

I toss. I turn. Alison comes in. "You're flip-flopping like a fish," she says. "You really have to pick a position and stay with it." I recognize the tone of voice. It's the one I use on my twins when they're throwing Play-Doh.

She takes my water away, and moves my iPhone so I can't check the time.

Finally, I drift off for about three hours of sleep. The results come in the next day: It worked. If I wear a CPAP machine, it virtually eliminates my snoring. Clearly, I'm going to need one eventually.

But can my combo-pack of pillows and nasal strips buy me a few years time before I order it? I need another test. I promise to make an appointment.

Falling Asleep Faster

I am watching *Dr. Oz*, as I do nowadays during those interminable minutes when I'm brushing and flossing. The man makes a good point. He says the phrase "falling asleep" is a misleading one. It makes it sound too passive. You have to work at going to sleep. Strategize. You have to attack the task. Maybe "jumping asleep" would be a better phrase.

I call up Dr. Michael Breus—a sleep specialist and author of the book *Good Night*—to get some tips. He had plenty—a shower, because it lowers the body temperature. Tart cherry juice, as it has melatonin, a chemical that regulates sleep. I should impose a curfew on myself, and turn off all TVs and computers an hour before bedtime.

But the sleep trick that worked best? Doing third-grade math problems. When I'm lying there, waiting to go to sleep, my mind usually resembles one of those shirtless perps on *Cops*, running all around, ranting and raving. A few years ago, I tried counting sheep, but it doesn't work. A 2002 Oxford study showed counting sheep actually delays the onset of sleep. They're just too dull to stop us from worrying about jobs and spouses.

Dr. Breus told me to try counting backward by three. I did. And in just a few seconds (400, 397, 394 . . .), I felt my a gear in my brain click to neutral.

Counting backward by threes is just challenging enough that it keeps my interest, and boring enough that it puts me to sleep. In a couple of minutes I'm out. I'm hoping it lasts, and that my mind doesn't become immune, like the morphing supergerms I keep reading about.

Sleeping Longer

There's also this sophisticated secret: I go to sleep earlier.

I'd always thought I could train myself to sleep six hours, wean myself off of the seven and a half hours I need to feel rested. That I failed and was always exhausted, I blamed on my own laziness.

Dr. Breus let me off the hook. He says everyone has a built-in sleep requirement. Usually from six to eight hours, though one World War 1 veteran was famous for only needing one hour.

You can't change your limit. It's not like playing golf or drinking vodka. It doesn't become easier with practice. If you don't get your allotted time, you're damaging your health and job performance.

I moved my bedtime from 1 a.m. to 11:30 p.m. It was an act of trust. I had to trust my future self that he would be more efficient tomorrow if I went to sleep now. I had to convince myself that sending postmidnight e-mails was counterproductive. Turns out I didn't trust myself too well. Most nights I was still up at 12:30 A.M.

I got better at sticking to my new bedtime after buying a gadget called the Zeo Personal Sleep Coach for $199. This is the DIY version of the sleep clinic featured in Tim Ferriss's book. You strap on a relatively unobtrusive headband before turning in. It measures your brain waves, and figures out how long you slept, and how well (the ratio of REM to light to deep sleep). Then the Zeo's algorithm calculates your nightly grade, or ZQ.

What the pedometer did to my walking, the Zeo did to my sleeping—it turned it into a game. I got competitive with myself. My first ZQ score was 44 (terrible), and after a week, I got it up to 68 (not bad). In good news for the publishing industry, reading a nonelectronic book for seven minutes before turning off the light seemed to boost my score, helping me go to sleep faster and deeper. Anecdotal, but still. Our industry needs all the help it can get.

Julie borrowed the Zeo and notched up 99 her first night. Nearly two hours of restorative deep sleep! I've never seen her so pleased with any accomplishment. "I *knew* I was a great sleeper," she said. "I need to enter a sleep competition."

Her mother nodded proudly. "She was the only baby in the world who slept through the whole night ever since she got home from the hospital."

Checkup: Month 19

Weight: 159
Average hours of sleep per night: 7.5
Average hours sedentary per day: 4
Chest press: 185 pounds (15 reps)
Health blogs read daily: 6

I'm doing okay, but my grandfather isn't. I brought Lucas and Zane to visit, and as soon as we enter, I can tell his health had gone south.

He is sitting in his recliner, his mouth more ajar than usual, his skin looser, his body more immobile. Without help, he can barely shift position.

"Is he frozen?" Lucas asks.

I blush. I try to recover by pretending Lucas was asking about the temperature, "No, he's not cold. The heater is on. I'm sure he's warm."

"He looks frozen," Lucas repeats.

Thank God my grandfather is hard of hearing.

My grandfather looks over and lights up, just a little. "What are you writing nowadays, A.J.?"

I tell him about the health book. Lucas picks up a green balloon in the corner. My aunt Jane tells me the physical therapist gave it to Grandpa. He's supposed to bat it around to keep moving.

"Put it back, Lucas. It's for Great-Grandpa."

"No, he can play with it," says Jane. "Play with Great-Grandpa."

Lucas swats the balloon to his great-grandpa, who swats it back. They thump the balloon back and forth, Lucas laughing, my grandfather smiling.

It's a trope that people become like children in old age. But there's nothing quite like seeing it happen firsthand. My grandfather's daughters—he has five, and one is always on hand—wipe his chin with a napkin when he drools. When his eyelids start to droop, they ask, "Who's a tired boy?"

Old age is a long, slow loss of control.

Infancy has no control either. I've always found it odd when people say "happy as a baby." Really? Sometimes it's fun, like when you get to see your parents do something witty, such as rip a piece of paper in half. But other times, babyhood seems terrifying. You're so reliant on others. You've got to howl and thrash and pray the mashed bananas will appear. The saving grace is, babies don't know what independence feels like. Old people know what they're missing.

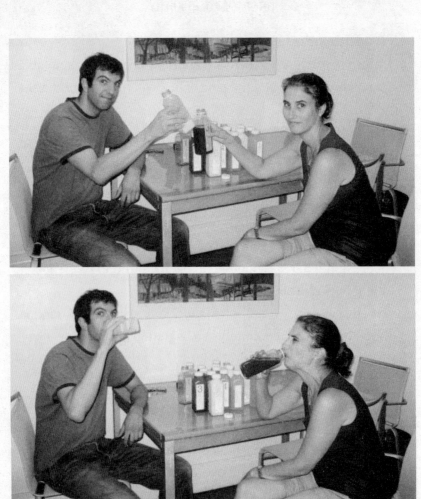
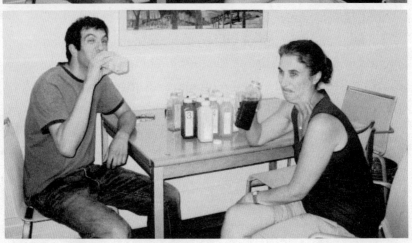

Chapter 20

The Bladder

The Quest to Figure Out What to Drink

I'VE SPENT A LOT OF time thinking about what to eat, but little on what to drink. This month, I'll change that.

I've ordered something called the BluePrintCleanse. This program is the juice fast of the moment, endorsed by a phalanx of women's magazines and a smattering of B-list celebrities (Elisabeth Hasselbeck and Julia Stiles.).

I ordered it online, and the next day a box arrived with thirty-six bottles, enough for my three-day fast. Actually, enough for both Julie and me. I've convinced her to go juice for juice with me.

The bottles come in five colors: light yellow (lemonade with agave nectar and cayenne pepper), white (cashew milk), green for veggie juice (celery, spinach, kale, etc.), red (apple, carrot, and beet, etc.), and dark yellow (pineapple juice, apple juice, and mint).

This juice is, quite possibly, the most expensive in the history of beverages. I'm hoping each one of those lemons in the spicy lemonade was caressed by a shiatsu masseuse while still on the tree. Because we're talking four hundred dollars per person.

In the morning, I give Julie her juice, and we tap our plastic bottles together. "Cheers!"

We each take a swig of the green one. Not bad. Sort of a fancy cousin to store-bought vegetable drinks, the pashmina to V8's cotton.

"What do you think?" I ask.

"It alternates between being refreshing and making me want to gag."

By 10 a.m., I'm a little hungry, but nothing painful. I go out to run some errands and come back an hour later. I find Julie in our bedroom. She's . . . chewing?

"What's in your mouth?"

Julie scurries away, giggling.

I chase after her. "Open your mouth!"

"Ahhhhh."

It's clean. Whatever it was, she'd swallowed the evidence. I let her off with a warning.

Time for the spicy lemonade. We tap bottles again, and take a swig. It's sweet, but with a cayenne pepper kick.

"What do you think?"

"This is so not my thing," says Julie. "I just really like food."

I spend the day at the library, reading my health books. I come home at 5 p.m. Julie is sitting in the living room, Lucas on her lap. He is in a post-tantrum stupor. She doesn't look much happier.

"I have a headache. I got half my work done. I am not happy. Frankly, I'm acting like a bitch."

I nod as noncommittally as I can.

"I'm having leftover Indian food."

So that's it for Julie. She made it nine hours into our three-day fast, not counting the cheating. Julie fasts on Yom Kippur, but that's her limit. The BluePrint people don't have thousands of years of guilt-tinged heritage behind them.

I keep on fasting for the next two days. In a dietary version of the Stockholm syndrome, I start to like the juice more and more, especially the almond milk, which is thick and yogurty. I can feel it sloshing around in my otherwise empty stomach.

I keep waiting for an epiphany. Some people say juice fasts clarify their thoughts and give them fresh energy. Unfortunately, for me, it's having just three effects.

- Hunger. I'm hungry enough that I started to salivate at the sight of lettuce. I repeat: lettuce.
- Crankiness. At one point, I called up BluePrintCleanse customer service because I thought they sent me the "Renovation" cleanse instead of the "Foundation" cleanse I'd ordered. I snapped at them. I turned out to be wrong. Which made me feel terrible. Can you imagine a grumpier clientele than underfed New Yorkers?
- Spaciness. On the third day, it took me nearly a minute to dial my phone, as I kept losing my train of thought.

When it was over, I craved something solid, something that could break a window if you threw it hard enough. I settled on a potato, which I roasted in our toaster oven, and which was wonderful and nonliquidy—though certainly not optimally healthy (too starchy).

It's been a week since my juice fast. I do miss that almond milk—that could have been one of the best beverages I've ever tasted. But do I feel clear of toxins? Not really.

Maybe I didn't go into it with an open enough mind. The problem for me, though, is there's little science supporting juice fasts. There's a bit of science on the benefits of general, intermittent fasting. According to a study by the National Institute on Aging, periodic fasting can give you the same antiaging results as calorie restriction.

But the cleansing claims? As Katherine Zeratsky, a registered dietician with the Mayo Clinic, writes in a cleanse-debunking article, "Most ingested toxins are efficiently and effectively removed by the kidneys and liver and excreted in urine and stool."

I don't think I'll be ordering a second round from BluePrint. Probably a relief to their customer service reps.

The Water Cure

The healthiest liquid, unless you are a newborn in need of colostrum, is, of course, the simplest liquid: water. Sugar-free, vitamin-unenhanced water. We were built to consume it.

How much per day? I'm sure you've heard we should be drinking eight eight-ounce glasses a day. It's a handy mnemonic, but turns out, it's based on flimsy or nonexistent evidence. The Mayo Clinic puts it this way: "If you drink enough fluid so that you rarely feel thirsty and produce between one and two liters or more of colorless or slightly yellow urine a day, your fluid intake is probably adequate." Which is good. I don't have to count ounces, one fewer item on my ever-expanding list of daily tasks.

Unfortunately, another question—what *kind* of water is healthiest?—turns out to be a surprisingly complex problem that took me on a fascinating quest.

First I learned that it's probably not the stuff that flows out of your faucets. My friend Charles Duhigg did a massive investigation of drinking-water safety for the *New York Times* in 2009. It was a disturbing series. "As many as 19 million Americans may become ill each year due to just the parasites, viruses, and bacteria in drinking water." Nineteen million. And that's just the germs. There's also carcinogens. "Some types of cancer—such as breast and prostate cancer—have risen over the past 30 years, and research indicates they are likely tied to pollutants like those found in drinking water." Even if the water passes EPA standards, it could still be problematic. Your water could be within legal limits for arsenic, but still pose the equivalent danger of 1,664 X-rays.

Dear Lord. I'd mindlessly drunk tap water all my life. I figured the government wouldn't let poison flow from the taps. But in general, I'm too trusting of the government. I'm the polar opposite of the Tea Partiers. I have no problem with a nanny state. But in this case, the nanny state has been chatting on the cell phone and ignoring the baby as it plays with matches.

Another option: bottled water. Global bottled water is a $60 billion business, as Elizabeth Royte wrote in her book *Bottlemania*. It's a decent alternative—but not necessarily safer than tap.

The regulations for bottled water are just as imperfect as those for tap. In 2006, Fiji ran an ad that said, "The label says Fiji because it's not bottled in Cleveland." Don't mess with Cleveland. The city had their water tested, and found no measurable arsenic. Fiji had 6.3 micrograms of arsenic per liter—below the legal limit, but still.

The other problem with bottled water—at least on the liberal Upper West Side—is the glares you get from neighbors. Carrying nonreusable bottled water is an environmental crime. As my friend told me, only half jokingly: "If you open an Aquafina water and listen carefully, you can hear the earth weeping."

So for my stress level, I'm looking beyond bottled water. I asked

Duhigg to point me toward the healthiest glass of water in New York City. "Go to Pure raw food restaurant," he says. "It's the only restaurant that boasts its filtration system on the menu."

I enlist Julie to come with me to the downtown restaurant. She's more than a bit skeptical about trekking forty-five minutes for a glass of water.

"This better be one hell of a glass of water."

"I hear that it's like the dew from God's front lawn," I assure her.

When we get there, the owner—Sarma Melngailis—a stunning, blond former Wall Street trader, tells me, about the Tensui Water Filtration System. "Everything in the restaurant is from this water. The vegetables are washed in it. Even the toilets have it."

Julie suggests a slogan: "Pure Food and Wine—where you can drink the toilet water."

Sarma laughs, though demurs. She does say she likes the water so much, she has her pitbull mix drink it as well.

The waiter pours us our glasses. I swish it around in my mouth. I chew it like an oenophile.

Julie takes a sip as well. Her eyebrows rise.

"It's actually really good."

"*Really* good," I agree.

I'd always thought drinking water tasted like drinking water. About as interchangeable as aspirin brands or Michael Bay movies. I was wrong. This glass of water was particularly smooth, like drinking velvet or riding in a Bentley. This was damn tasty water.

The Tensui system claims to suck out the contaminants (chlorine, fertilizers, pesticides) while at the same time "enhancing" your water with minerals (calcium, magnesium, zinc, potassium, negative ions, etc.), Though I should mention there has been little research on whether mineral-enhanced water is better for you.

I'd love to install the Tensui system in my home. The only problem? It's fifteen-thousand dollars.

I ask Duhigg what to do. He says the best brand that won't force me to take out a second mortgage is called PUR. They are water filters are just plastic pitchers with replaceable carbon filters inside. New York has pretty decent water, Duhigg adds. "If you lived in New Jersey, you'd need a more sophisticated system, like a reverse osmosis one."

I buy my PUR filter. To make sure it works, I hire a lab to test my tap water versus my PUR water. Sure enough, the PUR filter screens out arsenic and something called "trihalomethanes," which have been linked to bladder cancer. Of course, there's a catch. If I forget to change my PUR filter after two months, it'll start to leach chemicals into the water and poison my family.

Cold Comfort

One final water dilemma: What's the healthiest temperature of water?

Many of my books and advisers made a strong argument that tepid water is healthier. There are several alleged reasons: Tepid water soothes the stomach. It might even prevent cancer.

This was welcome news. For years, I've had an outsized aversion to iced water. I've always found it jarring and headache inducing.

So passionate was I about tepid water, I wrote a college essay about the man who foisted iced drinks on the world: Frederic Tudor, a nineteenth-century Bostonian known as the "Ice King." Tudor was a genius. He bought up eleven New England ponds, and during the winter, he chopped them into enormous chunks and shipped them south. Even smarter, Tudor created a demand where none existed. A wily PR man, he whipped up a vogue for iced drinks, promoting them in Cuba, Martinique, and the southern United States.

Tudor even makes a cameo in *Walden*. Henry David Thoreau was innocently trying to commune with nature and avoid paying taxes when Tudor's ice cutters descended on Walden Pond to carve it up. I resent Tudor and his misbegotten legacy of ice.

So I was delighted to hear that ice was dangerous. Until I researched it further. Unfortunately, evidence-based science gives no support to tepid-water claims. Most hard-nosed physiologists dismiss them as hogwash.

To my dismay, I've learned the opposite is true. Ice-cold water is probably healthier. Why? Cold water helps you lose weight. It has negative calories. Here's how Cornell psychology professor Brian Wansink explains it in *Mindless Eating*: "Since your body has to use energy to heat up an iced beverage, you actually burn about one calorie for every ice-cold ounce you drink. So that 32-ounce drink will take you 35 calories to warm up. No big deal? If you drink the recommended eight 8-ounce glasses of water a day, and if you fill those 64 ounces with ice, you'll burn an extra 70 calories a day."

Seventy calories. That's nearly the equivalent of walking a mile. Or according to my Fitbit, having passive sexual activity. So in the interest of my waistline, I've started putting ice in my portable BPA-free charcoal-filtered water bottle.

Checkup: Month 20

Weight: 158
Average grams of sugar per day: 25
Coffee cups per day: 1.5

Times unsuccessfully attempted to switch to green tea: 7
Number of yoga instructors who have been surprisingly rude
    to me: 2

Turns out fear of failure is a wonderful thing. It has inspired me to train for my triathlon every day. I alternate biking, running, and swimming.

I've convinced myself I know what I'm doing, thanks to my copy of *The Complete Idiot's Guide to Triathlon Training.*

When I pedal my bike around the Central Park's Great Lawn, I don't just push down with each leg. I do the full-circle pedal, keeping the pressure in all directions, down, up, forward, back. You know, like a triathlete.

When I swim in the Jewish Community Center pool, I roll my body from side to side. I slide my arm into the water like I'm putting on a coat—as opposed to slapping the water, which is what I used to do. Again, like a triathlete.

When I run, I do my grueling High-Intensity Internal Training. This Sunday, I came back to the apartment from a run. My face was red, a half-moon of sweat soaked the bill of my baseball cap.

"Welcome back," Julie says. "You missed a great show."

Lately, the twins have been staging the occasional off-off-off-Broadway show for Julie and me. They usually choose an improvised version of a fairy tale, like "Three Billy Goats Gruff." But the play itself is almost incidental. The important part of the production is the preshow announcements—that's what gives them the biggest thrill. Lucas will step in front of the couch and announce with great pride, "Ladies and gentlemen. Please turn off your cell phones."

Zane will add, "And no flash photography because it disturbs the actors."

Then they'll congratulate each other on a job well done, giddy from the glamour of theater management.

But today, I missed both the preshow announcements and the show itself.

"Can I see an encore performance?" I ask.

The twins shake their heads. They're not in the mood.

I hate missing these historic events. I'll live. I'll see another one of their plays, no doubt. But this underlines something that's become increasingly clear: The health project is taking time away from my family. Which is probably not healthy.

I recently read an article in the *Wall Street Journal* called "A Workout Ate My Marriage" about exercise widows and widowers. There are quotes from therapists who counsel couples in which one spouse's fitness addiction drives them apart. The men skip breakfast with the family for an early-morning trip to the gym. The women miss romantic dates in favor of doing laps at the Y.

The bottom line: Health obsession can turn you into a selfish bastard.

There are half solutions. Whenever I can, I try to exercise with my family. I run errands with Zane on my shoulders, or jog behind Lucas as he rides his Razor scooter.

And then there's this rationale: I'm exercising so I can be around for my kids when they get older. Maybe you need to be selfish in the name of selflessness.

Chapter 21

The Gonads

The Quest to Get More Balls

I'VE BEEN MEANING TO SEE a urologist since my ill-starred at-tempt to jump-start my sex life. Now fate—and *Esquire* maga-zine—have led me to Harry Fisch, M.D.

I meet Fisch at an *Esquire* symposium where he's giving a lec-ture on men's health. A prominent urologist—a regular on the *Dr. Oz* show and author of *The Male Biological Clock*—he's six feet tall and has good posture, sharp suits, and a big laugh. He exudes his favorite hormone, testosterone.

After his lecture, I approach Fisch and tell him I'd be interested in coming to see him. Fisch says absolutely.

"When I do a prostate exam, it's easy. I use one finger. Maybe two if I need a second opinion."

He unleashes his big laugh. "I love that joke. Heard it from a cabdriver."

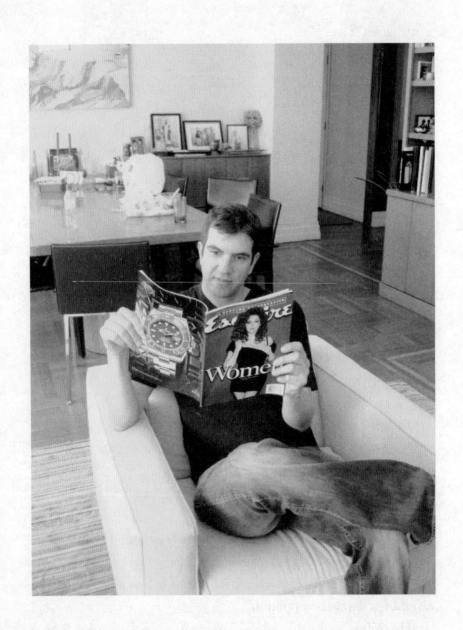

A week later, I'm in his sleek Park Avenue office, sitting across from him at his desk.

"The penis is the dipstick of the body's health," says Fisch. "What's good for the heart is good for the penis. It's all the same blood vessels. Should we do a checkup? C'mon, let's do a checkup."

We walk to the exam room next door, and I drop my pants as Fisch snaps on a glove. As he examines me, I turn my head and look off into the distance, sort of like Obama in that Shepard Fairey poster. It's my attempt to retain a smidgen of dignity.

Fisch stands up. He's not going to sugarcoat it.

"You have old-man testicles, my friend. Low-hanging fruit."

The problem, he says, isn't just aesthetic. It's that these may be a sign of low testosterone.

"You came in and thought you were healthy," he says. "You're not. I mean, you're fine. But you could be a lot healthier. It's about prevention. Twenty years down the road, you'll be like this." Fisch slopes his shoulders and shuffles along.

Before we decide on a course of action, Fisch says I should get a semeanalysis.

"Okay. Who should I call to set one up?"

"How about now?"

Turns out, there's a lab right next door and they have an opening. I was unprepared, but it's hard to say no to Fisch.

At the lab, the technician gives me a cup and leads me to a small room. Maybe it's my low testosterone, but this room seems like the least erotic place in the world. I don't think all the maca powder in Peru could help me here.

I shut the door—and am alarmed to find out the walls are far from soundproof. It's probably my imagination, but the walls seem to amplify the sound, as if there are woofers and tweeters hidden in there. I listen as the staff chatters away about delivery times and appointment switches. I notice a small table loaded with a stack of *Playboys*, which is thoughtful, I suppose. But these *Playboys* are faded and wrinkled, dating back to an era when Hugh Hefner didn't need Pfizer's help to have sex.

It took a while. I'll skip the details, but let me put it this way: I was in there so long that when I emerged, the guy at the lab said, "Congratulations."

A few days later, Harry called.

"Your testosterone is low!" he says.

His tone was so confident, almost upbeat, which made me unsure how to react. My testosterone clocks in at 245. The average for a man my age is 300 to 1,100.

Low testosterone sounds bad, and embarrassing. But on the other hand, so what? What's the problem with being a little on the, shall we say, artistic side. I'm not looking to join the New Zealand rugby team.

Fisch says low testosterone can cause cardiovascular problems down the road. It's also linked to fatigue, depression, and decreased muscle mass. Here's how Fisch writes about it in his book: "Men with levels below 300 ng/dl (a condition called hypogonadism) tend to have little interest in sex and are usually nonconfrontational, socially inhibited, and physically weak. They are also often very intellectual, creative, expressive, and likable." The intellectual and creative part sound good. The socially inhibited, not so much. "Men with higher-than-normal testosterone tend to be just the reverse: Obsessed with sex, competitive, aggressive, extroverted, physical and tending toward more action-oriented activities or careers." A mix would be nice.

How'd my testosterone get into such a sorry state? Several factors play into it:

It's partly genetic, of course. But your testosterone level drops when you get married. It drops again when you have kids. It drops every moment after your thirtieth birthday—men lose about 1 percent of testosterone a year. (Though estrogen increases, "which is why we get man boobs," says Fisch.) It drops when you have too much fat, especially abdominal fat. (I'm still working off my stomach.) I also have a vein-related problem down below called "varicocele."

The good news, says Fisch, is that there are natural ways to boost your T. First, a healthy diet: walnuts, salmon, whole grains, the usual suspects. I've been eating this way for months, so I can't rely on that. Fisch says that moderate exercise helps. Extreme exercise doesn't, which is why, according to Stanford professor Robert Sapolsky, professional soccer players have lower-than-average testosterone. I've been exercising moderately for months, so I've got that covered.

"I once read that you can boost your testosterone just by holding a gun," I tell Fisch.

"That's true, but that's just a temporary fix," he says.

He says we should think bigger: supplements.

There's a long history of men trying to turbocharge their testosterone. Even before scientists discovered the chemical testosterone, they knew that the testes had more than a little to do with manliness. In the 1920s, a French surgeon named Serge Voronoff made a fortune with his "rejuvenation" techniques, which were rather extreme. He grafted chimpanzee-testicle tissue onto the penises of men. He promised a longer life, a higher sex drive, and better eyesight. Another doctor offered the same procedure with goat testicles. You'd pick your goat, much like you pick your lobster at a restaurant today, writes Pope Brock in his book *Charlatan*. Amazingly, none of the animal transplants worked as promised.

Now we have a more scientific wave of rejuvenation techniques. Thousands of men take testosterone supplements, either with gels, creams, or injections. The promises remain the same, except for the better eyesight part. The questions about treatments' efficacy remain as well. Data are mixed. Some studies show testosterone shots increase muscle mass and energy. Others—including a major study published in the *Journal of the American Medical Association* in 2008—indicate that men taking testosterone did not improve in mobility, strength, or quality of life.

Skeptics also say we don't know the long-term effects. One doctor I talked to said that the current trend of testosterone supplements reminds her of the hormone replacement therapy trend in the 1990s. Millions of menopausal women underwent HRT to combat low libido and energy, only to find out later that it raises the risk of breast cancer and heart disease.

Fisch says he's not doing testosterone replacement therapy. He calls it "testosterone *normalization*." He recommends against the testosterone gels and creams for me. I have children, and if I hold my kids against my gelled-up chest, the testosterone could rub off. Next thing you know, Jasper needs to borrow my Gillette Mach3.

Instead, Fisch recommends a drug called Clomid. This will make me produce my own testosterone. Oddly, this drug is usually used by women to boost fertility, but it also works in men to increase hormones called FSH and LH, which spur testosterone creation. Also, Clomid resets your baseline testosterone level, so you don't have to keep taking it the rest of your life, Fisch says.

When I get home, I tell Julie.

"What are the side effects?" she asks suspiciously.

"Well, it'll increase my sex drive."

"I think your sex drive is just fine."

"There's a chance it'd increase my baldness."

"That's not good."

I tell Julie many doctors are leery, seeing as the science behind it is new, and we don't know all the side effects yet.

"No, I think it's a bad idea."

"I should at least try it."

"No, don't do it."

She shut me down. So for a week, I didn't pursue it. Which I thought was appropriate, in a way: You can't get much more testosterone-deprived than having your wife forbid you from taking testosterone supplements.

But in the end, I defied my wife, just to see what a higher testosterone level can do. I start popping 25 mg of the chalky-white pill every day.

The blogger Andrew Sullivan wrote a story in the *New York Times Magazine* several years ago about his experience of injecting synthetic testosterone to counteract the effects of HIV. For him, it was like a magic potion that transformed him into a Nietzschean Übermensch. His energy, confidence, and libido exploded.

My transformation is more subtle. If Sullivan's testosterone shots were a double espresso, my pills were a mild chamomile tea. Since I began taking them two weeks ago, I do feel slightly more energetic. My three miles on the treadmill at the gym seem easier. I don't get the postlunch hunger for a nap.

And yes, my libido is higher. The sexual thoughts bubble up even more relentlessly than usual. I try to read *Esquire*, since it's my job and all, and I get sidetracked by a photo of a Barcelonan model named Claudia Bassols. She seems interesting. She was in a film with Jean-Claude Van Damme and has been a judge on *Iron Chef*. I should probably check out her website, as an *Esquire* employee. Thus commences ten minutes of clicking through her photos.

I'm not allowed to give details of Julie's and my sex life, but I'll say this: We are definitely ahead of the Japanese average.

Am I more aggressive? Well, the other day, I'm on line at the subway station to buy a Metrocard. There are three Metrocard machines, but a single line that feeds into all three. Everyone's taking their turn. It's civilized.

Then this guy in a charcoal suit walks right up to the machine on the left, cutting all eleven of us on line.

"Excuse me," I say. "There's a line here."

"The line's only for those two machines," he says, pointing to the other two.

"Really?" I say. "You're really going to cut all these people?"

He pecks away at the keypad. I'm not just annoyed, I'm furious. What a selfish liar.

"I can't believe what an asshole you are. I mean, I hear about people like you, but I rarely see it in person."

I'm not the confrontational type, so my words are startling even to me. The other people on the line look at me with what seems like a mix of gratitude, embarrassment, and nervousness.

The line-cutter makes some response, but I can't hear it, perhaps because the blood is pumping in my ears. Plus my hands are shaking. That can't be good for me.

I'm guessing the T had something to do my uncharacteristic rage. There's clear scientific data that links testosterone and aggressive behavior. But, of course, I never underestimate the placebo effect. Especially when it comes to my slightly higher energy and confidence. It turns out the evidence linking those to testosterone is flimsier.

A few weeks later, I take another testosterone test. When the e-mail with the results pops up in my in-box, I don't want to click it. What if I'm lower? But I man up and open the document. Yes!

Four hundred sixty-five. I'm higher, and in the normal range. I am officially masculine. After two months of pill-popping, my testosterone rose to 650, which, I told Julie, is somewhere between lumberjacks and Italian prime ministers.

But it occurs to me, maybe this is the worst time in history to be upping my testosterone. As Hanna Rosin points out in *The Atlantic*, perhaps modern society is better suited to women. "For the first time in American history, the balance of the workforce tipped toward women, who now hold a majority of the nation's jobs . . . The attributes that are most valuable today—social intelligence, open communication, the ability to sit still and focus—are, at a minimum, not predominantly male. In fact, the opposite may be true."

So maybe I should be taking estrogen supplements instead. In fact, I recently read a study that women's language skills are at a peak when they are ovulating and the estrogen levels are highest. So maybe estrogen injections would make me a better writer.

For now, I'm going to get off the Clomid. In part, because I'm sick of checking my temples to see if I'm getting balder.

Checkup: Month 21

My grandfather's back in the hospital, this time because he's having trouble breathing. I take a cab up to visit him.

"Oh, the hospital," says the driver, when I told him the address. "Hey, what's the difference between a doctor and God?"

"I dunno."

"God doesn't pretend he's a doctor."

What is it with taxi drivers and doctor jokes? I smile politely. I'm not the best audience for Borscht Belt comedy right now.

I board the elevators filled with low-talking visitors and get out on the ninth floor. I make a right at the flower display, and a left at the end of the hall, and end up in room 134.

There's my grandfather. He's lying on his right side, propped up by three pillows. He's got a white-and-blue hospital robe, an oxygen tube under his nose, and eyebrows as bushy as ever.

His mouth is open in an oval shape and his lips seem to have all but disappeared.

"Look who's here!" says his daughter Jane. She's slept here the night before in her blue tracksuit. "All these visitors are better for you than antibiotics!"

"Hi, grumpy Grampa," I say. He breathes heavily and shallowly and looks at me through half-lidded eyes. He lifts his hand about half an inch—it seems so small and limp now, almost ladylike—and I take it in mine. He squeezes my fingers. Or maybe that was my imagination. I can't tell.

Jane is holding a stick with a moist cubic green sponge on the end, and is dabbing it around his mouth to keep him moist. She leans over and kisses his cheek.

Bloomberg business channel plays on the television. A businessman till the end.

I feel like I should try to entertain him. That's my job. So I tell him stories about my sons and my work. I tell him about my *Esquire* interview with George H. W. Bush, during which the former president said, off the record, that a certain politician's wife had a "pickle up her ass." I tell him in a loud and upbeat voice, because Jane says he responds better that way.

He doesn't laugh, but he nods slowly, and his big eyebrows twitch a bit.

The hospital gown doesn't cover his legs, which are red and yellow, veiny and sausagy. I hate those gowns.

My sister, Beryl, knocks on the door and comes into room 134.

Her face goes a little white when she sees his body, which seems so shrunken. "Hi, Grandpa," she says, shakily. "How are you doing?" She then excuses herself to go to the bathroom. A couple of minutes later, she comes back red-eyed.

"The foliage is beautiful nowadays," says Jane. "We have to get you out of here so you can enjoy it."

Grandpa doesn't say anything. Just keeps breathing loudly.

Is he really going to get out of here? It's that crucial balance between delusional optimism and realism. I get out my laptop and show him some videos of our family, including one of Beryl's daughter playing a mouse in a musical based on *The Wind in the Willows*. She looks so purposeful in her red hat and red coat, gazing off into the horizon as she sings.

A doctor comes in to inspect the rash on his arm where the IV enters.

Another knock on the door, this time his longtime secretary, Valerie. "Hi, Chief!" she says. Her friend is with her, and wonders if she could say a prayer. She clasps his hand and asks God to help heal this man. Does my grandfather understand what is going on? What does he, as a lifelong agnostic, think of the prayer?

As I leave, I tell my grandfather, my voice as chipper as I can manage, "I love you, Grandpa. I'll see you soon!" He tries to say something, but it just comes out as a moan.

He died two days later. There was some sort of delay at the hospital, so my late grandfather's body lay there for six hours on the bed. A strange fate for a man who was always on the move.

Marti told me, "He looked so calm and peaceful lying there, it was hard to remember that he wasn't just taking a nap."

We held the funeral for my grandfather at a West chester cemetery on a sunny and brisk day. There were only fifteen of us gathered around the grave, just the immediate family. A public memorial would be held later.

A little black amplifier rested on top of the pink headstone. One by one, we came up, picked up the mike, and said our goodbyes as the wind rustled the red leaves on the tree behind us.

We talked about his civil rights work. About his love of family, justice, apple cider, and *Alice in Wonderland.* About his trips to Ghana and the time LBJ grabbed him by the lapels for a photo op.

Marti read a letter he wrote that showed he was a sucker for silly word games: "This letter is being written without a salutation, since you know who you are and it is silly therefore to tell you who you are. And to call you dear when everybody knows you are very cheap."

After the speeches, four cemetery workers lowered the coffin into the ground with thick straps. Most of the family walked to the nearby grave of my late aunt to pay respects. But a couple of us stayed behind, including me and my cousin Rachel, a psychology student from Baltimore.

We picked up the two shovels stuck handle up in the pecan-colored dirt. We didn't talk. Rachel began by tossing a shovelful of dirt onto the coffin. It landed with a soft thud.

I bent my knees and tossed in a shovelful, as well. It thudded, and the dirt skittered across the coffin.

We needed something useful to do. We needed to have a purpose, even if that purpose was pointless since the workers would do it if we didn't. Or maybe it wasn't. Maybe Grandpa would have appreciated it. One last show of affection from his grandchildren. It felt like tucking someone into bed for the last time.

We worked silently as the dirt made a collection of mounds on the coffin. I was bending deep at the knees, putting my back into it. Every shovelful a heaping one. This work was physical, and physical felt good right now. I was starting to sweat under my suit. Grandpa was not a man who did things half-assed. Neither would I.

The next day, the *New York Times* ran an obituary of my grandfather. It was the obituary he would have wanted. It called him a "peacemaker," which is a pretty great noun. It talked about his passion for resolving conflicts, quoting an old *New York Times Magazine* article that said, "Some men look at Gina Lollobrigida and are set aflame. Kheel gets the same reaction by exposure to a really tough strike situation."

And it made him sound like James Bond. "Even though Mr. Kheel handled disputes for bakers, garbage collectors, plumbers, subway conductors, tugboat captains and undertakers, he was an unabashed bon vivant, fond of fast sports cars and fine food."

The photo showed him holding two phones, one pressed to each ear, in the middle of a negotiation between labor and bosses—maybe the bus drivers' union, maybe the symphonies'. It didn't say, and it didn't matter.

Julie clipped the obituary and pasted it onto a piece of cardboard, which I thought was a lovely, nostalgic gesture in these digital times.

There was a short video on the *Times* website. They must have interviewed him just a couple of years ago, and he must have known it was a pre-obituary Q&A. They filmed him, gray-haired and still articulate, against a black background.

"How do you want to be remembered?" he is asked.

My grandfather laughs. "I don't want to be remembered," he says. "I want to stick around for a while longer."

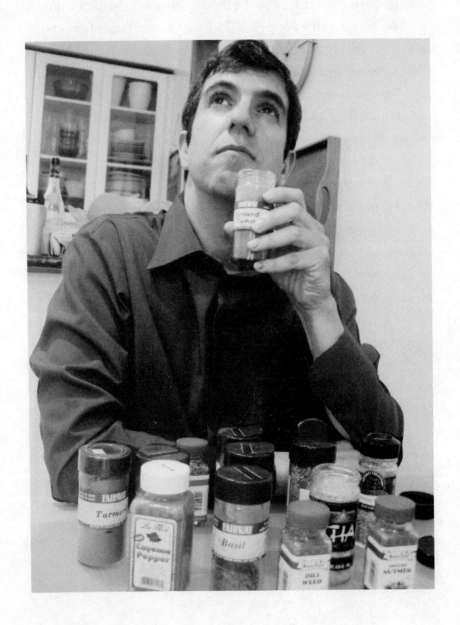

Chapter 22

The Nose

The Quest to Smell Better

IT'S BEEN TWO WEEKS SINCE the death of my grandfather, and I'm eating too many refined carbs. I'm barely exercising, feeling fatalistic. I keep going back to the Jim Fixx argument, that chestnut of defeatist reasoning: Whatever I do, I'm still going to die, so why waste all this time and energy? And it's not like my grandfather consumed a strict diet of cruciferous vegetables. Why should I?

I'm bingeing. I'll eat a handful of raisins, peanuts, and chocolate. Then a granola bar with twenty-four grams of sugar. And more of the trail mix. Then I have the bag in my face like a farm animal. I recently read a brilliant description of bingeing. The passage isn't even about eating, but it was the best portrayal of a shame spiral I've ever come across. It is from Plato, and describes a man who walks by a heap of corpses. The man tries to look away, but then gives in and says to his eyes: "Look for yourselves, you evil wretches, take your fill of the beautiful sight!"

That's the way I feel about my stomach. It's a separate beast. "Here, you evil bastard, have your Fig Newtons and shut up."

I need to snap out of it. A few weeks ago, I'd set up an appointment at the Monell Chemical Senses Center in Philadelphia. This is America's biggest research facility devoted to studying human smell and taste. People are always telling me to "smell the flowers." Maybe that's what I need to do.

I take the train down to Monell on a snowy Tuesday morning. It's hard not to spot the center, thanks to the entryway's giant bronze sculpture of a nose. It's probably a good thing the same designer didn't work on the Harvard Urology Center.

The eighty scientists at Monell believe that smell and taste are an underappreciated part of healthy living. It's why I came.

Smell and taste have been tied to health for millennia. The earliest doctors diagnosed with their nose, as Esther Sternberg points out in *Healing Spaces*. The scent of sweet urine meant diabetes, for instance. And now that's coming back into vogue thanks to a field called "olfactory diagnostics," which analyzes some of the thousands of compounds we exhale in every breath.

It's long been suspected that smell and taste influence mood and behavior. Florence Nightingale believed the scent of lavender relaxed her patients. In Civil War hospitals, she would anoint the foreheads of wounded soldiers with the floral fragrance. Unfortunately, until recently, there's been little rigorous research on the topic. Instead, we've gotten the fuzzy-headed but well-meaning field of aromatherapy. Aromatherapy—the use of scented essential oils—isn't bad, necessarily, especially if accompanied by a foot rub. But it's about as scientific as numerology.

The Monell Center is out to fix that.

One of Monell's scientists, an energetic woman with blue glasses named Leslie Stein, gives me a tour of the six-story building: microscopes, truck-size freezers, mazes for mice, a dozen white lab coats hanging in a row, scientists crunching data in their offices, skullcaps with electrodes, an Oscar the Grouch doll in the children's testing room. Oddly, it's not a smelly building. I could only detect one researcher's microwaved moo shu chicken.

There's a sense of adventure here. Smell isn't nearly as well researched as any of the other senses. "I love it because it's uncharted territory," says Sweden-born researcher Johan Lundström. "Whenever I have an idea, I can design an experiment to see if it's true, because chances are, no one's done it before."

Among the experiments Monell is conducting:

- Treating post-traumatic stress disorder, which can be triggered by odors such as the burning of explosives.
- Regrowing nerve cells. The nose's nerve cells have the unusual ability to regenerate after thirty days. Can doctors cause this regrowth to occur outside the nose?
- My personal favorite: an experiment that showed men's body odor has a calming effect on women. Which is a brilliant excuse not to shower. "Just trying to put you at ease, dear."

During my day at Monell, I'm given a variety of tests. For one, a researcher named Chris puts on a blue surgical glove and waves a series of eighteen Magic Marker–size pens under my nose. I have to choose what the pens smell like from a list of four options.

Is pen number five leather, turpentine, or rubber? I shut my eyes and inhale. It smells like my dad's loafers. Leather.

Another smells like honey. Then peppermint and anise.

The pens are convincing—enough so that I'm salivating, especially at the lemon ones. Pen number sixteen, on the other hand, is a repulsive fish smell that makes me jerk my head back.

I move on to taste, with a psychologist named Danielle Reed. I swig three dozen tiny vials of clear fluid, each one a different cocktail of sweet, sour, bitter, salty, and umami. The last is the oft-overlooked fifth basic flavor, sometimes called savory. It's a meaty taste found in shiitake mushrooms and fermented fish.

Dr. Reed now flips through the six-page answer sheet, studying my scrawled answers and the words I've circled from such lists as "soap, musk, urine, milk, and vanilla."

"Well," says Dr. Reed, looking up from my test. "You're our worst subject ever."

I chuckle. A wry sense of humor, these scientists. She is straight-faced.

"Really?"

"Yes. Really."

Apparently, I made some embarrassing mistakes. I confused sour for umami and semisweet for very sweet. I mixed up lemon and orange. I was their worst subject out of dozens who have taken the test over the years.

This is disconcerting. I never thought of myself as a gourmand, but to have the least discerning tongue in America—or at least of those tongues tested? Especially after I thought my discernment had improved, thanks to my cutting back on salt and sugar.

Once again, this whole health project is proving to be an exercise in radical humility. Contrary to what my mother told me, I'm not always above average. I'm not always Einstein doing physics or Michael Jordan playing basketball. And in some cases, I'm not even Michael Jordan playing minor league baseball during his ill-advised career switch.

The problem is, my chemical senses aren't just dull. I'm blind to certain smells and tastes. I have trouble tasting umami, for instance. And I can't smell something called "androstenone."

I'm not alone. Fully 45 percent of Americans are genetically incapable of sensing androstenone. It's a steroid that occurs in sweat, urine, and, oddly enough, pig saliva. Apparently it smells quite rank. I will never know. So enjoy that sweaty odor, you lucky bastards in the 55 percent of the population.

There's a lot of variation in our abilities to taste and smell, much of it genetic. I had no idea until today that I am essentially smelling and tasting a different world from my friends.

Despite my low scores, I didn't leave the Monell Center in a funk. The situation isn't totally hopeless. I can take action. The scientists made two additions to my to-do list: sharpen my sense of smell, and use odors to help me relax. I'll explain them in order:

Experiment 1: Sharpen my smell

"There is an association between our ability to smell and our mental health," says Dr. Pamela Dalton, a researcher at Monell. "It's not a perfect correlation. But people who lose their sense of smell show signs of depression."

She tells me that keeping your sense of smell sharp could help keep your brain healthy. "Exercise it like you would any other muscle."

And what makes for a good odor workout?

"Go to your spice rack, and try to identify the bottles without looking."

That's my new favorite game. Julie hands me a bottle, I keep my eyes shut and take a deep sniff.

The first few times, everything smelled like nutmeg.

"Nutmeg," I say.

"No, turmeric," says Julie.

"Nutmeg," I say.

"No, lemongrass."

And so on. But I've done it twenty times now, and I'm scoring about 50 percent correct.

My nose is improving. I'll likely never learn to smell androstenone. But I can become better at identifying the scents my nose already knows. As one Monell researcher explained it to me, "You can't make your car go faster, but you can become really good at obstacle courses."

The average person smells about ten thousand odors, at least according to Nobel winners Richard Axel and Linda Buck. Nobody's quite sure. Unlike taste, it's not a relatively simple matter of five basic flavors. It's a complex, not-fully-understood system that, we think, involves nasal receptors recognizing the different chemicals' shapes.

However it works, I find I'm noticing a lot more smells out in the world—both for good (the sweet potatoes at the corner restaurant) and ill (the smell of chlorine that permeates the local Jewish Community Center).

I've also noticed that enthusiastic smelling has perils. When I met a friend for lunch and took in too deep a draft of air, he looked at me suspiciously and said: "Are you sniffing me?" Kind of.

Experiment 2: Relax

The olfactory part of the brain is tucked into the ancient section, the so-called lizard brain, which means it is tangled up with the emotions. Smell can bring on powerful feelings, as anyone who has read Proust's books or at least his Wikipedia page knows.

Which smells and which emotions? Depends on the individual.

Aromatherapy goes wrong here, say Monell researchers. Aromatherapists make sweeping statements like "vanilla will relax you." But it depends on experience.

"You can't say 'lemons are invigorating,'" says Stein. "If you grew up walking through a lovely garden filled with roses, you'll have positive feelings when you smell roses. But if you are first exposed to the smell of a rose at your grandmother's funeral, it's the opposite."

Dalton, for instance, says the smell of diesel puts her in a happy mood. As does a lemon-rose scent.

"I travel a lot," says Dalton. "And when I'm in an anonymous hotel room, falling asleep can be an issue, so I bring a safe odor with me." (Wisely, she goes with lemon rose instead of diesel.)

My scented sedative of choice: almond. Maybe it was the marzipan that my dad always brought home. Who knows? But the scent of almond makes stress melt away and lifts the mild depression.

Inspired by Dalton, I've started carrying a small bottle of almond oil next to the Purell and miniature fork in my pocket. I unscrew it on the subway and inhale a few nostrilfuls. Passersby probably think I'm huffing glue, but I'm too relaxed to care.

Checkup: Month 22

Weight: 159

Average minutes of self-massage per day: 4

Average hours of sleep per night: 7

Meals incorporating cinammon (which can increase insulin receptivity): 1 in 3

My nose adventure was helpful. I'm back to my spinach salads, my meditation, my modified Bass Method. If I squint, I can see the project's finish line off in the distance; I'm trying to finish in two years, for the sake of my sanity and my publisher's.

I'm not free of morbid thoughts, though. One of my big preoccupations is this: What if it's all for naught? What if my DNA has doomed me, and I have some hidden disease that will strike me dead before year's end?

This anxiety inspired me to spit into a skinny tube and send it off to a lab in California.

I just got back my results this month. The proper reaction would be gratitude to my parents for bestowing upon me relatively decent DNA.

There are no huge problems. I have a slightly elevated risk of having a stroke, arthritis, and restless legs syndrome. I'm hypersensitive to warfarin blood thinner. But overall, the test says I'm free of huge risk factors for horrible diseases.

So gratitude would be appropriate. Instead, I keep focusing on one result. That I have gene marker rs174575, Genotype AA. Which means, according to the testing service's website: "Being breastfed raised a person's IQ by an average of six to seven points."

I was not breast-fed.

Therefore my IQ is six to seven points lower than it could be. At least in theory. This news is disturbing. Six to seven? That's not a trivial amount. Imagine what I could have been like. Maybe my Netflix queue would be filled with Truffaut films instead of Albert Brooks movies. Maybe I'd read *The Mahabharata* in its original Sanskrit. Maybe I'd be decoding genomes myself instead of sending my drool out in a FedEx box.

What do I do? Do I mention this news to my mother and give her a guilt trip? It's hard to blame her. In her day, formula was seen as breast milk's equal, if not its superior.

Perhaps I should compensate. Watch more Yale literature

classes on YouTube. Buy a calculus textbook. On the bright side, my slightly lower IQ means I probably have worse recall. Maybe I'll soon forget I have a depressed IQ.

I'm also trying to remember this is far from gospel. I went with one of the most reputable consumer services—it's called 23andme. com—but genetic testing in 2011 is still in its infancy. Think of it as better than tarot cards, but much less reliable than X-rays. It has a long way to go before it's considered an accurate diagnostic tool.

The problem is, there's rarely a one-to-one relationship between a gene and a trait. There's no single "you will go bald" gene. It's dozens of genes, interacting with one another and the environment. It's going to take a while to put this jigsaw together.

Services such as 23andme do give some results that you can act upon immediately to improve your health. This is especially true with the information about your sensitivity to medications. But mostly, for now, it's more about curiosity and potential future knowledge.

That will change. In a few years, genetic testing will be a massively important health tool, yielding tons of useful information. If we have an elevated risk for lung cancer, we can avoid secondhand smoke. We will be able to tailor prescriptions.

This tidal wave of information will come with its own complications. There will be a whole class of information that we can't act on. Diseases for which there is no known cure. Vulnerability to environmental factors—like the breast milk—that are too late to fix.

I just read a great but scary book, *Origins* by Annie Murphy Paul, about the many ways gestating infants are affected by the mother's behavior. Poor Julie. My sons will come to know all sorts of things she did wrong while pregnant. "You breathed unfiltered New York air? What were you *thinking*?"

DNA testing will present us with a Tree of Knowledge problem.

On the whole, I think I would bite that apple of full bodily knowledge. I'd like access to unlimited information, despite the perils.

I'd asked Julie to send in her spit to 23andme as well, and she agreed. Again, we got lucky. Aside from higher odds of heroin addiction, which has yet to be a problem, she's relatively free of risk factors.

We called the genetic counselor together to make sure we hadn't missed anything. She assured us, no, Julie's genes looked okay.

"I do want to ask about one result in her DNA," I say.

"Yes?" asks the counselor.

"I'm interested that she has rs1800497," I say. "It says people with this genotype are much less efficient at learning to avoid errors."

"Well, it's only got a single star next to it, so that indicates it's a finding we have the least amount of confidence in."

"But it IS interesting," I say. "Do you think she's not efficient at learning from mistakes?" For instance, Julie keeps deleting episodes of *The Office* before I have a chance to watch them.

"My husband's trying to bait me," says Julie.

The counselor stays professional. "It's from just one study is with twenty-six Germans. It's really too small a sample to have a lot of confidence in the data." At this point, she says, rs1800497 is more for curiosity than actual valuable data.

"Well, it's interesting is all," I say.

After we hang up, Julie asks me if I have a gene for being a schmuck.

Chapter 23

The Hands

The Quest for Magic Fingers

I JUST FINISHED READING a 1980 book called *Hands* by Princeton professor John Napier. It's a lovely work. A mix of anatomy, history, and lyrical odes to our fingers, it's a classic of hand literature (a genre that's bigger than you might think). And it has made me a convert. Consider this sentence alone: "Visitors at the zoo indulge in transports of delight at the way an elephant reaches for an apple with its trunk . . . but give not a moment's thought to the ineffable capabilities of their own hands."

He's right. We take our hands for granted, unless you happen to be a stoned college sophomore staring slack-jawed as your palm opens and closes. Most give all the glory and attention to the brain and the heart. We view them as our body's CEO and president. The hands? We dismiss them as mere interns.

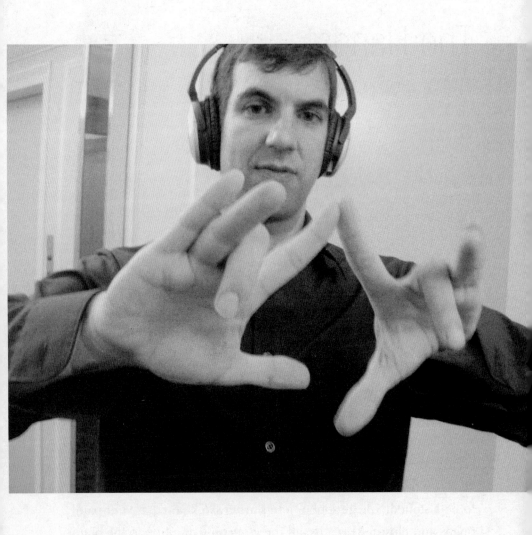

Not me. If my goal is total body health, I can't overlook this gorgeously complex package of twenty-seven bones and thirty muscles. I will heed Napier and try to improve the ineffable capabilities of my own hands. I will have the strongest, nimblest hands I can.

The benefits might be surprising. George Washington University neuroscientist Richard Restak writes in his book *Think Smart*, "Since no part of the body is more functionally linked with the brain than the hands—with larger areas of the brain devoted to the fingers than to the legs, back, chest or abdomen—developing nimble finger skills is a surefire way of improving brain function."

Another pro-hand book—*The Hand: How Its Use Shapes the Brain, Language, and Human Culture*—argues that we have it all backward. The brain isn't king. The brain is the hand's handservant. We evolved our complex frontal lobes—at least in part—to allow us to manipulate our fingers. Meanwhile, philosopher/motorcycle-repair-shop-owner Matthew Crawford—the author of *Shop Class as Soulcraft*—says that modernity's alienation can be blamed on manual incompetence. When we lost our ability to replace a light switch and whittle a block of wood, we lost our souls.

If you want the healthiest hands, you've got to talk to a man named Greg Irwin. He calls himself "the Richard Simmons of hands, but without the shorts." An Ohio-based musician and salesman, Irwin has a blond goatee and a wide, friendly face. He is the inventor of a grueling aerobic workout for the hands called "Finger Fitness." You can find his videos on YouTube. If you watch them, please don't be offended. In the intro to one, Irwin warns: "I do not feel that social gestures should restrict the smooth flow of the gestures in this video. Therefore, none of the positions you see in this video are meant to have any social meaning."

And then he flips you the bird.

Thanks to Napier, I know that the middle finger—or "obscenus"—got its naughty rep because "the longest digit is ideally disposed to carry out indelicate scratching operations."

But as Irwin says, giving the bird in his video is nothing personal. It's just part of a workout in which you extend and stretch all the fingers. Irwin's handwork is remarkable to watch. His hands blur as the fingers cross, weave, pop, do the Vulcan salute and the heavy-metal devil horns. It's a digital ballet.

I set up a private video lesson with Greg on Skype. Several weeks ago, Greg had sent me a starter kit that included two DVDs and a pair of apricot-size silver Chinese therapy balls. I'd been meaning to practice, but I've been too busy washing vegetables, running laps, and sniffing my spice rack. "Let's start with the basics," he says. "Bend, fold, tap, press."

I put my hands in the prayer position, bend them right, bend them left. Then I stumble. Which way do I fold them again?

Greg isn't impressed. "You've had my video for weeks and you can't do the bend, fold, tap, press?"

I sheepishly admit that's true.

"Well"—Greg softens—"you're probably a little nervous doing it in front of me."

Also true.

I love Greg's passion. He eats, sleeps, and dreams hands—and sits in them as well. His home has four hand-shaped chairs. In fact, Greg's house is packed with the world's largest collection of hand paraphernalia—hand-shaped cups, hand-shaped flashlights, hand-shaped jewelry—not to mention the purple handprints that decorate his bathroom walls.

He invented Finger Fitness nearly thirty years ago. He was studying music at college (incidentally, he helped develop the first electronic xylophone) and working as a dishwasher. During a break at his job, he started playing the air piano. Inspiration hit.

Skeptics often ask him why it is so important to work out the hands. His answer: to avoid injuries, to prevent arthritis, and to allow us to live our lives in peak condition. "We're all small muscle athletes," says Greg. "Think of how this world would change if we all did Finger Fitness. People would type faster. Surgeons would do operations faster. McDonald's would make change faster. Older people could button their shirts."

Greg has sold thousands of DVDs—many to musicians and athletes. He's even appeared on *The Tonight Show with Jay Leno*.

But he's frustrated. "I'm dumbfounded this hasn't caught on more. I've been doing this for years. I feel like I have the next peanut-butter-and-chocolate. And I can't even get my own mom to do the exercises."

The exception, he says, is China, which he visits several times a year. "They get it over there. Healthy hands, healthy mind."

I feel for Greg. I was about to type "My heart goes out to Greg," but realized that's just another instance of cardio fetishism. No, my hands go out to Greg. I promise him I'll spread the news about Finger Fitness in my book. I pledge to do five or ten minutes a day while waiting at red lights or watching TV. Greg says he will let me know about the results of an upcoming Finger Fitness study at Winston-Salem State University.

"The hand is really devalued in Western society," he says. When he shows his hand tricks at parties, snooty intellectuals often dismiss it as a mere gimmick. "This might sound out there, but I almost think the mind is threatened by the hands," says Greg. Or as comedian Emo Philips once said, "I used to think the brain was the most wonderful organ in the body. Then I realized who was telling me that."

Holding Hands

I've made another discovery: I shouldn't keep my hands to myself. Holding hands is healthy. A study by James Coan, a professor of neuroscience at the University of Virginia, brought sixteen married women into his lab, and subjected them to the threat of electric shock while he studied their brains on an fMRI machine. He found that holding the hand of your husband reduced the stress. Even holding a stranger's hand calmed the women's brains, though not as much.

I've been on a mission to hold Julie's hand as much as possible to reduce my stress level. (Strangers' hands, not so much. To me, the health benefits are outweighed by my fear of microbes and getting punched in the face.) I've been clasping Julie's hand a lot: as we walk, as we talk, as we watch TV.

I'm surprised how much I like it. I'd forgotten how good human contact can be, even if that contact isn't in bed and goal-oriented. When we lock fingers, I visualize an fMRI glowing in my brain's happiness nooks and crannies.

At first, Julie liked it, too. I even got a few "Awwws." But she has limits. When I tried to hold her hand during a fight over how to discipline our kids, she pulled away like I was a patch of poison oak.

"It'll lower our stress level during the fight," I said.

"I want to be stressed during the fight. That's the whole point."

My sons are less discriminating. I better take advantage now, while they still let me. It's a shame that male hand-holding is socially unacceptable in America (though not in the Middle East). Holding Jasper's little hand on the way to school is such a joy, fleeting though it may be.

Typist's Cramp

Thanks to Finger Fitness, my hands feel more dexterous and stronger than ever. Julie even complimented my skills when we attempted to tie plastic lanyard bracelets for the boys. If my upcoming triathlon included origami, I'd be set.

Ironically, though, this chapter has taken me a bit longer to type than usual. I switched my typing style after talking to Dr. Michael Hausman, a noted hand surgeon in New York.

Hand and wrist aches are more common than ever. New hand maladies pop up every day: Wikipedia lists BlackBerry thumb, Rubik's wrist, Cuber's thumb, stylus finger, and my favorite, Raver's wrist, which you can get from repeatedly waving a glow stick in the air (see, kids, ecstasy really is bad for you).

Steve Jobs hasn't helped. The new fad for touch screens has caused problems, including swiper's finger, and whatever you want to call the cramps people get from pinching the images bigger and smaller.

But the most common cause is probably typing. "You remember the carriage return?" says Dr. Hausman. "The carriage return was your momentary rest. Now you just type on and on page after page with no pause and that causes lactic-acid buildup. I tell people they should get those annoying digital watches. And every ten minutes, have it beep. And then shake your hands."

I took Hausman's advice. Every ten minutes, my iPhone goes off. I have to set to the "slot machine" sound so I get a momentary dopamine spike before I realize I haven't won any money, and remember to shake my hands.

I don't think I'll continue the ten-minute alarms. Studies show that distraction is unhealthy. Lack of focus can cause depression and stress. In this case, I'm going to screw my hands.

This means I may be at risk for a repetitive stress injury. But at least I won't get carpal tunnel syndrome, which is a separate malady that involves the squeezing of the nerve in the wrist. Despite common misconception, carpal tunnel is mostly inherited, says Hausman. One of the only activities that seem to be associated with carpal tunnel is using a vibrating power tool in a very cold room. "It showed up in people who were processing human cadavers—cutting off limbs for orthopedic use." Hausman adds: "Jeffrey Dahmer was probably at high risk for carpal tunnel."

Checkup: Month 23

Weight: 158

Miles walked while writing: 1,144

Push-ups till exhaustion: 167

Potatoes eaten per week: 2 (trying to eliminate, since many
  nutritionists think they cause weight gain)

My triathlon is in two weeks. I've convinced my trainer, Tony, to join me, so that he can share in the triumphs, humiliations, and lactic-acid body aches.

I'm training every day. Also worrying every day. Mostly, I'm terrified of the arctic water, a long time phobia. I have spent hours scouring the Internet for ideas on how not to become hypothermic. I found the world's only electronically heated wet suit. It's got two graham-cracker–size lithium batteries sewn into the neoprene. Could work. In my risk assessment, electrocution is better than freezing. But it costs a thousand dollars, so Julie put the kibosh on it.

I've had to settle for plan B. I've rented my neoprene booties, my neoprene skullcap, and my full-body nonelectronic wet suit. I took them all for a test swim in the JCC pool. As I walked out of the locker room, I got some quizzical stares. Was I a Navy SEAL on a mission to assassinate one of the white-haired women in the Aquafit class?

I slid into the pool feetfirst. Unfortunately the water was eighty degrees, which won't help me toughen up. Regardless, while I was there, I figured I'd do some laps. I started my crawl. A fiftyish man switched lanes to get farther away from me. "Your outfit is making me uncomfortable," he said. Which gave me a macho thrill.

In nontriathlon news, I got an update on the Jack LaLanne interview. Today his publicist left a voice mail.

"I'm sorry about this, but Jack has to postpone because something has come up."

Ugh. I've already bought my tickets and made my hotel reservations. He can't honor his commitment? What kind of a man is he? Something better came up, did it?

I dialed the publicist, ready to snap at him.

"What happened?" I demanded.

"Jack's got health problems. It doesn't look good."

"I'm sorry to hear that."

"Yeah. Really not good."

"Oh."

"Things are shutting down."

I'm simultaneously ashamed of my pettiness. I'm stunned that Jack LaLanne is going to die. Jack LaLanne passing away? That doesn't compute. He said it himself many times, "I can't die. It would ruin my image."

But the publicist wasn't lying. A few days later, I read on CNN. com "Jack LaLanne, fitness guru, dies at 96." There he is, a photo of him in his blue jumpsuit, his arms raised in the "check out my guns" pose, beaming.

First my grandfather, then LaLanne. Two vibrant men in quick succession, both gone at ninety-six.

I do an Internet search for "Jack LaLanne and Dying," and find this quote: "I train like I'm training for the Olympics or for a Mr. America contest, the way I've always trained my whole life. You see, life is a battlefield. Life is survival of the fittest. How many healthy people do you know? How many happy people do you know? Think about it. People work at dying, they don't work at living. My workout is my obligation to life. It's my tranquilizer. It's part of the way I tell the truth—and telling the truth is what's kept me going all these years."

In honor of Jack, I head off to the gym to work at living.

Chapter 24

The Back

The Quest to Stand Up Straight

MY LOWER BACK HURTS. Which doesn't make me particularly noteworthy. I'm one of 65 million Americans with back pain, nearly as many as voted in the last presidential election. Back pain is the single most common reason people visit the doctor.

My backache is mild. It usually kicks in at the end of the day. But as I age it'll get worse, especially with my posture.

What a disaster, my posture. I amble around looking like Hominid Number Three in those evolution charts. Partly, it's out of laziness. But partly, it feels odd to me to thrust out my chest, almost presumptuous. During my biblical year, I learned that the Talmud suggests that we *not* walk in a jaunty, upright manner. Be humble in your posture, it says. Stooped shoulders were a sign of respect. So when my posture is criticized, I explain that I'm honoring my forefathers.

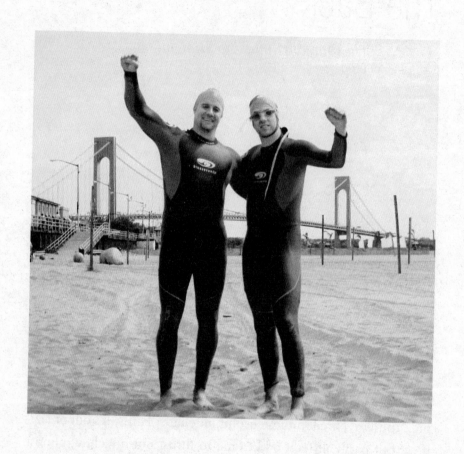

Unfortunately, bad posture exacerbates back pain. It puts pressure on the discs, and can also cause neck problems and knee problems. I need a spinal makeover.

When I comb the Internet for posture experts, I find a guy named Jonathan FitzGordon who was profiled in the health section of the *New York Times*. His website says he teaches yoga, but he's most famous for his walking lessons.

FitzGordon came to my apartment the next week. I'm not sure what I expected an official Walking Instructor to look like—perhaps Phileas Fogg in *Around the World in 80 Days*, a fastidious Brit with a crisp bowler who said "Spit-spot!" John was not that. He's a burly, sweatshirt-clad forty-eight-year-old who grew up in Brooklyn. He retains a bit of an accent.

"Do you have any experience with walking?" FitzGordon asked.

Um, yes? A little? I didn't want to come off as too cocky, but the truth is, I've been walking for quite some time—decades even.

FitzGordon slipped off his shoes and observed me as I stood, then as I walked across my living room. If it's possible to cluck your tongue with your eyes, that's what FitzGordon did.

His verdict: I'm a sloucher. My pelvis juts too far forward, my shoulders lean too far back.

I shouldn't feel too bad. I'm just a typical American. Thanks to our sedentary lifestyle, Americans don't know how to walk and stand correctly.

FitzGordon fishes a photocopied cartoon out of his bag. It's Robert Crumb's famous "Keep on Truckin'" illustration, the one with the blue-suited man leaning so far back while walking, it looks like he's lying on an invisible La-Z-Boy. That's America's problem. We lean too far back.

"Walking should be falling forward," says FitzGordon. That's the way we were built. "Go to the playground, kids walk leaning forward. They turn their motor on." FitzGordon walks across my living room with his body angled forward, like Wile E. Coyote about to break into a sprint.

The key is to stick your butt out, says FitzGordon. Kim Kardashian has the right idea.

"See how Julie is standing with her pelvis tucked under?" FitzGordon says.

Julie has taken a break from work to join us in the living room. I'm not sure she expected a critique of her pelvis.

"Release it, Julie. Stick your butt out."

She tries.

"More. More. Nice."

Julie, her rear protruding, is giggling. She says she feels like Mrs. DeLauria, her sixth-grade teacher, who was famous for her steatopygic figure.

But FitzGordon is pleased. "Moms tell their daughters, 'Tuck under.' Women feel like, 'I'm walking in the street, I'd better hide my stuff. I say, you better *strut* your stuff.'"

I try to strut. I walk past the couch with my butt extended, my body leaning forward, my arms dangling. "I feel kind of like a monkey," I say.

FitzGordon lights up. "That's exactly what I'm looking to hear. Go ape, young man! That's one of my main phrases." Gorillas have flat lower backs, so they can't lean backwards.

I look at Julie and give a faux-humble shrug, as if to say, "Who knew I'd be the teacher's pet!" Julie gives me a faux smile.

I ask John what he thinks of traditional posture advice. It's a mixed bag, he says.

Balancing the book on your head is a good idea. "You want to lengthen the back of the neck," he says. On the other hand,

"There's no worse instruction in the world than to have your shoulders back." When your shoulders are back, your breath gets shallow. You want to breathe from the stomach.

After FitzGordon left, Julie and I spent the next few days trying to walk in the FitzGordon way.

We agree we like the standing-up-straight part. "Posture!" we'd say to each other as we passed in the kitchen. With my back straight, I felt more decisive, more confident, like I'm an admiral of a midsize navy. There may be a reason for the phrase "get some backbone."

I ordered the kids around with decisiveness. "Please do not touch my computer," I'd intone. And they'd back away, practically saying "yessir, yessir." Would that have happened if I were slouching? Perhaps not.

I also loved FitzGordon's suggestion of walking with shorter steps. It made me feel more efficient. It made me speed up. If there's one thing I've learned in my experiments: The body affects the mind. The quicker the step, the quicker the mind.

But as for the butt protrusion, it still feels odd, no matter how many times Julie and I do it. We stick out our burns, but within a few minutes, our bums have edged forward.

To make sure Julie and I were on the right track, I called up a more traditional back expert, Dr. Jeffrey Katz, Harvard professor and author of *Heal Your Aching Back*. His posture advice? It wasn't as detailed as FitzGordon's. Basically, don't overthink it. "There really isn't a lot of evidence-based medicine about posture." AstraZeneca isn't funding a lot of posture studies. The best we know is just to stand up straight and lengthen the back. So for now, at least, I feel better about ignoring the protruding butt.

In his book, Katz gives suggestions on relieving back pain, which I've road tested as well.

- Neck exercises. You should press your palm against your forehead for ten seconds. It's sort of an extended "oy gevalt," which is appropriate, because that's the way I felt when I found out I'd have to be doing another set of exercises (hands, legs, neck—I'm over an hour a day).

- When sitting at the desk, keep your butt as far back in the chair as possible. A good reminder for both Julie and me, who sit like flour sacks.

- When lifting, bend the knees and keep the back straight, then push with the legs. This technique I knew about. But had I done it? Not really. It's a revelation, an immediate relief from pain. I've started to avoid rounding my back in any situation. If I have to talk to Lucas about an important *Yo Gabba Gabba!* plot point, I squat down next to him, then I bounce back up. It cuts the usual I'm-an-old-achy-man feeling in half.

Squatting Revisited

I've become quite the squatting enthusiast, it seems. Which would make John happy. He, and a surprising number of other people, believe we should all be squatting at bus stops and while eating dinner, as did many Asians of previous generations. There aren't many studies on it, but I'll bet it's better than sitting. Almost anything is better than sitting.

The first time I tried squatting for a few minutes, I was in pain. I told Julie it felt like my legs had menstrual cramps. She found the description odd.

Turns out, I was doing it wrong. To do the proper "Asian squat," you have to keep your feet flat, your legs spread wide, and your arms forward for balance.

I tried it at a bus stop after taking Jasper to school.

"There's room," said a man in a Yankees jacket, sliding down the bench to make more space.

"No thanks. I prefer squatting."

He nodded stoically.

After a month of walking tall and squatting low, my back does feel better. The pain has receded to the occasional twinge. I still sometimes walk like a monkey, but mostly to scare the kids.

Checkup: Month 24

Weight: 159
Dogs petted: 12
Minutes singing per day (possible stress reliever): 10
Days practiced didgeridoo: 2

This month was the triathlon. Here's how it happened: My alarm chirps at 3:30 a.m. on a Sunday. My stomach feels leaden, since I'd carbo-loaded the night before. According to my research, prerace carbo-loading has little scientific benefit. I didn't care. I've been fantasizing for weeks about devouring a huge plate of linguine Alfredo, and I wasn't about to let snooty science get in my way.

I take a subway downtown to the ferry terminal. Tony is waiting for me, and we wheel our bikes up a ramp and onto the 5:30 a.m. boat to Staten Island. There are two types of passengers on that boat. It isn't overly difficult to tell them apart. There are those with lightweight bikes and aerodynamic helmets and water bottles. And there are those with leopard-skin skirts and primary-color hair and thick mascara, teens returning from a hard night of partying in Manhattan.

"I've just got one question," Tony says as we sit down in the ferry's main cabin.

"What is it?"

"Why?" says Tony. "Why do people do this to themselves?"

"You mean . . ."

"Why do they punish themselves by doing triathlons?"

I'm not sure what to say.

Tony and I are seated across from a thirtysomething man leaning on his Cannondale bike. He has a thin red beard and thick quads.

"That's quite a bag," he says, nodding at my duffel.

"Thanks," I say.

I believe I'm getting my first triathlon trash talking. Admittedly, the duffel—which was the only one I could find in our apartment—wouldn't have been my first choice. It was camouflage, but for reasons unclear to me, the camouflage wasn't the traditional green. It was made up of bright pink and red splotches. Which I suppose would be helpful if you're doing a commando raid on a nine-year-old girl's bedroom, but wasn't so helpful when you're trying to look like a triathlete.

"It's big, too," says the bearded guy. "You got another body in there in case yours gets tired out?"

Tony turns to me. "I'm not sure I like this guy's attitude."

Tony, the former parole officer, could lay this bozo flat with one pop to the mouth. But I tell Tony we have to save our energy for the race.

After disembarking, we knew we'd arrived at the right place. Speakers blared Bruce Springsteen's anthem to exercise, "Baby, I Was Born to Run." The field is covered with hundreds of bikes propped up on long steel bars. Helmets, towels, packets of blackberry energy gel are scattered everywhere. I hooked my bike onto the bar next to a twentyish blond woman zipping up her wet suit.

"Have you done this triathlon before?" I ask.

She nods.

"How's the water temperature?"

"Oh, you'll panic. You'll hyperventilate."

A few minutes later, on the line to the bathroom, I ask another veteran racer, a man with orange goggles perched on his head. "Oh, you'll panic. You'll hyperventilate."

We line up on the beach nearby, and at the whistle we wade into the dark Raritan Bay.

The icy water slides down the back of my wet suit and up my sleeve. It's unpleasant, like swimming in a Slushie. But . . . here's the strange thing. I don't panic and I don't hyperventilate. It's not that I'm particularly manly, despite my now-average testosterone. It's just that I had built up the ice swim so much in mind, the sixty-degree reality seemed manageable.

Maybe my calming techniques helped: I did my stomach breathing. I lay on my back. I cursed, since I know that this scientifically cuts down on the pain. I tried some Buddhist distancing: "Now, this is an interesting sensation on my skin!"

I splash along in the choppy water, popping my head up every thirty seconds to get oriented. Eleven minutes later, I curve around a spherical orange buoy and headed to the beach. All that angst for eleven minutes.

I run dripping to my little plot of land to strip off my wet suit. Here's one thing I didn't realize: how much of a triathlon involves wardrobe changes. It's like a strenuous version of a Broadway musical. After I peel the wet suit, I towel off, put on bike shorts, socks, shoes, and suntan lotion. It is a ten-minute production.

"Phase two," Tony says as we mount our bikes.

We pedal along a car-less road. It's been shut down for the race. We pass drugstores, a couple of dentist's offices, a field with a half-dozen turkeys. We zip through delightfully meaningless red traffic lights. We ride in silence.

Though the silence is broken by frequent calls of "On your left!" Which means some man or woman hunched with their chin on the handlebars whooshes by.

Thirty-three minutes and two sugary blackberry energy packs later, we dump our bikes off and start jogging on a boardwalk by the beach.

"I'm not in any hurry," Tony says. "So don't feel the need to sprint on my account."

"I don't have plans either," I say.

We plod along without a word. I've got a rhythm going—one inhalation for every four steps, one exhalation for every four steps. I'm tired, but not exhausted. I think I may make it. I trained enough—overtrained, in fact. As I say, fear of public humiliation is a great motivator.

I watch the water lapping against the piers. I listen to the cheering bystanders. "Almost there!" says a bald guy who already finished the race and has joined the crowd. I don't even mind his mild condescension. I'm kind of liking this. I'm finally feeling what Chris McDougall calls "the joy of running." I finally have the answer to Tony's prerace question: "Why?"

We cross the finish line and give each other a bro hug. We walk down a wooden ramp back to our bikes. Tony turns to me: "We did it."

And I say two sentences that, even as I was saying them, sound strange issuing from my mouth: "It was kind of fun, no? I'd do it again."

On the ferry back, Tony and I try to figure out whether the triathlon was, on balance, healthy or unhealthy. There were many unhealthy things about it. First of all, there was the postrace pancake breakfast, at which everyone (including me) shoved his or her face with simple carbs. There was also the lack of sleep, the noise, the three mouthfuls of microbe-filled New York Staten Island beach water that I swallowed during the swim, the unknown toxins from the Magic Marker with which our number was scrawled onto our hands and legs.

On the other hand, it had its healthy parts. It spurred me to exercise every day. And as for the pancakes, at least one of my fellow triathletes offered me sugar-free syrup, which is marginally better than Aunt Jemima's. It allowed me to socially connect with Tony, and for a few weeks there, I had a purpose, however absurd.

When I get home, I drop my pink camo bag in the hall and engulf my sons in a hug. "Did you win?" asks Zane.

"Well, I beat a lot of people," I say.

He seemed pleased.

"But I lost to hundreds of others."

That he didn't like.

(Note: This was not last triathlon I signed up for. A couple of months later, I paid a hefty, nonrefundable entry fee for the New York Triathlon. I'd be swimming nearly a mile in the Hudson River, biking twenty-five miles, and running six. Training was going well, I was feeling confident. And then, two weeks before the race, Tony sent me this e-mail:

Did you see that there was a fire at a sewage plant on 125th Street? Five million gallons of raw sewage spilling into the river every hour until they fix it. The city is urging all New

Yorkers to avoid contact with Hudson River water. I beg you to reconsider.

He didn't have to beg too hard. There's the thrill of a challenge, and then there's 200 million gallons of human waste. (I'm currently signed up for next year's triathlon.)

Chapter 25

The Eyes

The Quest to See Better

I LOVE WATCHING THE DISCOVERY CHANNEL documentaries on the body. They're so delightfully boosterish, they make me feel proud of this heap of bones and sinew. The narrator sells you on the human body like he's Ron Popeil hawking the latest vegetable chopper. "The eyes can see one hundred million colors! They can focus from infinity to inches in a fifth of a second! In complete darkness, they can detect the light of a single candle fourteen miles away!"

Which really are astounding statistics.

Unfortunately, my eyes aren't quite as astounding as the ones advertised. They're flawed. I'm nearsighted and have astigmatism. Which isn't compatible with my goal of being the healthiest man in the world.

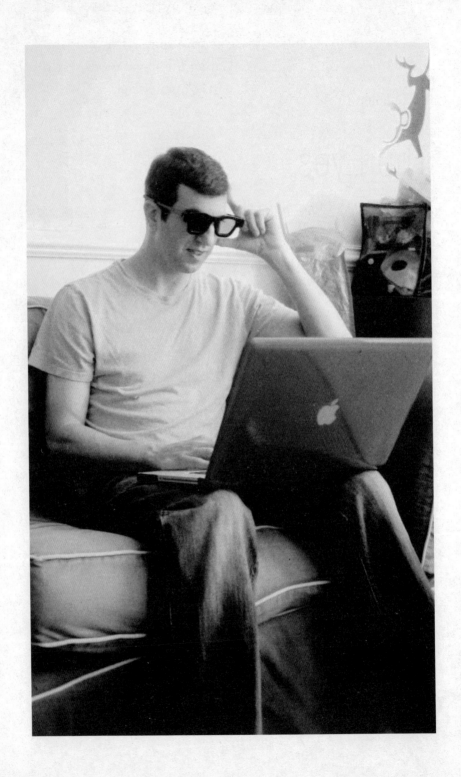

I've been trying to put some positive spin on my eyesight. In the past few weeks, I've been scouring the literature in search of advantages of myopia. One study says glasses wearers are perceived as more intelligent and are thus more likely to get hired. No less than 40 percent of people would wear fake glasses to land a job. So careerwise, I'm in good shape. (The study was conducted the College of Optometrists. It probably won't be published in the *JAMA* anytime soon.)

I also read that my flawed vision might boost my so-far-nonexistent art career. In *A Natural History of the Senses*, Diane Ackerman writes about how Cezanne's fuzzy still lifes and landscapes were partly the result of his poor vision. (His doctor commanded him to wear spectacles, but apparently Cezanne refused because he didn't trust medicine.) Degas had even more optical woes. He was both nearsighted and extremely sensitive to light, one of the reasons he might have preferred indoor's scenes to landscapes. If Degas's eyes had been stronger, we might have been looking at clear sunsets instead of his wonderful, clear ballerinas.

So that's something, right?

To get a more professional opinion on eye health, I consulted Dr. Peter Odell, affiliated with New York Presbyterian–Cornell Medical Center. My last eye exam was an appalling six years ago. He gave me the usual "which is clearer: this-or-that" tests. I also got the peripheral vision test, where I had to spot floating yellow dots. ("Just think of yourself as a pirate," said his assistant, Lynn, as I put my face against the black eye patch. "The fun Disney pirates. Not the Somali pirates.") I got the eyedrops that forced me to type my notes onto my computer in movie-poster-size type. The conclusion: I'm still nearsighted.

I asked Dr. Odell how to have the healthiest eyes and avoid

eye diseases. They are alarmingly prevalent. According to the *New York Times*, eye diseases—mainly glaucoma, cataracts, and macular degeneration—affect 10 percent of America. Twenty-six million people suffer from cataracts alone. And as the population grays, those numbers will climb.

Dr. Odell told me:

- Fruits and vegetables, of course.
- Fish such as salmon and tuna that are high in omega-3s may help prevent macular degeneration.
- Don't worry if you read in dim light, cross your eyes, or forget to wear your glasses one day. These are mostly harmless in the long term (though dim light can cause eye strain in the short term).
- Wear UV-blocking sunglasses. They are like Coppertone for the eyes.
- If you see floating black spots, flashing lights, or wavy lines while reading, get yourself to a doctor.

I met with another eye specialist, Dr. Paul Finger, and asked him the same question.

"Don't become a glassblower," he told me. Glassblowing emits infrared radiation and dust particles that can lead to blindness.

"Helpful."

"And don't be a boxer. They have a lot of detached retinas."

"What about sticking crochet needles into my eyes."

"Probably avoid that as well."

Sight Improvements

This is all solid advice on how to keep my eyes from deteriorating. But what about *improving* my sight? Making it sharper? Can I do that?

One option is Lasik surgery, which I'm still mulling. But I recently met one of the inventors of the Lasik technology, and guess what? He still wears glasses. He's wary of taking the risk. That gave me pause.

Lasik aside, there are several possible eyesight helpers. Here are the three most promising: cockiness, video games, and eye aerobics.

First, cockiness. In 2010, Harvard psychologist Ellen Langer conducted an intriguing series of experiments that she wrote about in *Psychological Science*. Her conclusion is that when you *believe* you can see better, you *do* see better. It's not as odd as it sounds. Scientists have long known that vision isn't just a matter of the eyes relaying info to the brain. It's a two-way street. We help construct the world with our brain.

In one of Langer's experiments, subjects read eye charts. Some were traditional, with the big *E* at the top. Some were reversed, with the big *E* at the bottom. The subjects looking at the reversed chart got better scores on the tiny lines than did those looking at the normal chart.

Langer and her team argue, this happened because subjects *expected* to be able to read the top line.

This experiment could explain the popularity of those quacky eye exercises on the Internet, the ones that promise you'll be able to ditch your glasses. (Make a figure eight with your eyes! Now focus on your thumb, then the wall, now the thumb!) Maybe these programs don't improve your eyesight. But they make you *believe* you're improving. And that false confidence leads to real gains.

Second, video games. A University of Rochester study showed that playing first-person-shooter video games made subjects 58 percent better at distinguishing contrast. They could detect shades of gray better. This improvement has real-world implications. Contrast sensitivity is crucial in night driving, for instance. I added video games to a file I have in my computer called "Healthy Vices," a list that already includes naps, booze, chocolate, and leaving the bed unmade, since dust mites thrive in the bedspread's heat and humidity.

And finally, I found a computer class called Vizual Edge. The military and a handful of pro sports teams (the San Diego Padres and the Houston Astros, among others) use this program. The idea is that with practice, you can improve your tracking and focusing and depth perception. Unlike other eye exercise programs, Vizual Edge doesn't promise to cure your nearsightedness, just to upgrade the speed and accuracy of your sight. They have studies to back up their claims. In a 2010 Texas A&M University study of college baseball players, Vizual Edge trainees were better batters.

"It's like weight training for the eyes," says Dr. Barry Seiller, a Chicago-based ophthalmologist who invented the program. The hope is you'll hit more home runs, catch more Hail Marys. Legend has it, Ted Williams could read the label on a spinning record. That'd be the windmill we're aiming at."

So I start my regimen of pumping pixels. Three times a week for twenty minutes, I don Vizual Edge's 3-D glasses—they're the old-fashioned kind, with one lens blue and one lens red—and try to spot floating arrows and rings on my computer screen.

I've also been playing my Top Gun video game; and telling myself I have bionic vision. And I am seeing better. At least according to my highly rigorous tests—the Snellen eye chart I downloaded from the Internet.

I made the mistake of telling Jasper that video games might be good for his vision. Now every time I try to shut down his Super Mario game, he has the predictable response. "But it's making my eyes stronger!"

I respond that his eyes would be better served by being outside. As Sandra Aamodt and Sam Wang write in *Welcome to Your Child's Brain*, kids' eyes need sunlight. Artificial light makes it much more likely they'll become nearsighted. Jasper responds to that by continuing to play Super Mario.

Checkup: Month 25

Weight: 158
Errands run per day: 4
Chews per mouthful: 11

I'd planned to stop Project Health after two years, but the goal line keeps receding. I still have body parts to revamp and self-experiments to try. The other day, for instance, I saw a *Dr. Oz* episode that recommended konjac root for suppressing appetite, and I add that to my monstrous to-do list. It's like when I want my sons to eat their dinner. "Just one more bite. Okay, one last bite. Now, last, last, superfinal bite."

I have to stop, or I'll go to my death trying to be the healthiest human. Next month is my last, last superfinal month.

I'm glad I didn't finish yet, though. Because a few days ago, being in good shape—and maybe having improved vision—came in terrifyingly handy.

Julie, the kids, and I were walking in the park on a sunny Saturday afternoon. Well, Julie and I were walking. The kids were zipping around on their scooters.

I got a cell-phone call from my dad. He wanted to meet us at a playground. I was giving him directions—I couldn't have been distracted for longer than twenty seconds—and then I look up. Zane and Jasper had vanished.

We were near the Great Lawn, a huge field filled with baseball diamonds and sunbathers. The path forks in front of us.

"You go that way, I'll go this," said Julie. She and Lucas hurried off to the left. I dropped the canvas bag with Jasper's baseball bat— I'd pick it up later—and started running to the right. Sprinting.

I was devouring that road. I sprinted by strollers and carts selling Popsicles and Gatorade. I jumped over puddles and dodged waddling toddlers. "Jasper!" I shouted. "Zane!" My newly strengthened eyes scanned for their orange scooters. "JASPER! ZANE!"

My adrenaline was pumping so high, I could have run across Manhattan, over the bridge, and into New Jersey. I understood the old legend of the woman gaining superhuman strength to hoist the car from her pinned children.

"Jasper! Zane!"

Then the magical thinking started kicking in. I started to conjure up all the horrible scenarios. The secret dungeons they would end up in, the screeching tires of a taxi that was about to run them over . . . and then I reined in my thoughts.

The fear was overwhelming. I was being sucked in. I chose anger instead. I could deal with anger. I was angry that my sons took off without looking back. I was angry at myself for being momentarily distracted. I was angry that there's not yet an affordable LoJack system for locating kids. We have the technology!

I sprinted around the entire Great Lawn at what I swear was Usain Bolt speed, no thought of slowing. "Jasper! Zane!" Four minutes and still no sign. I kept running.

And there, at the bottom of a path, near a statue of Shakespeare,

I spotted their orange scooters and their cute, worried little faces. They'd gone up to a police officer to tell her they got lost. Thank God, thank God, thank God.

I want to borrow the cops' handcuffs and latch my kids to my wrists until they are fifty-four years old.

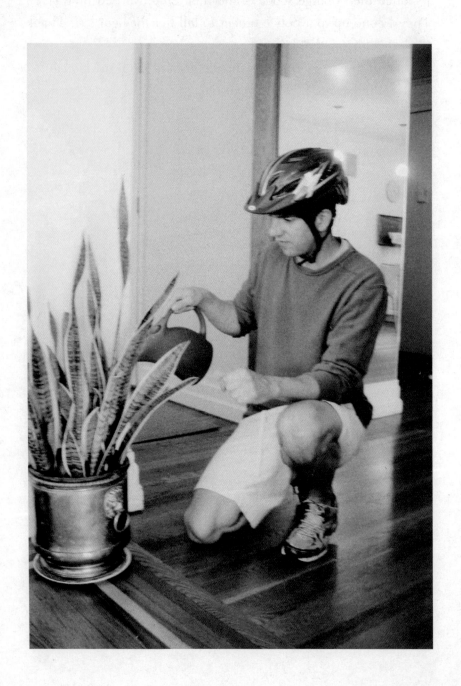

Chapter 26

The Skull

The Quest to Not Be Killed in an Accident

I JUST SPENT A TRULY harrowing half an hour reading the CDC's index of ways you can die and get injured. It's a mind-blowing document. Thousands of categories. They list the classics, like car accidents, of course. But also balloon, snowmobile, and animal-drawn vehicle accidents. They list dog bites, but also unpleasant contact with sea lions, macaws, and giraffes. There's accidental gunshots, but also rogue sewing machines and can openers.

It all makes you want to curl up in your bed. Except that your bed could kill you in any number of ways.

- entanglement in bed linen, causing suffocation (category T71)
- fall while climbing into bed (W13.0)

- burns from highly flammable sheets, spreads, pillows, or mattres (X05)
- drowning involving bed (W17.0)

I'm not sure how the mechanics of bed-drowning work, even with a water bed, but that's what's fascinating about this list. Half of the causes I wouldn't have conceived of on my most paranoid day. Like Y35.312: hitting a bystander with a baton.

The point is, you can eat your Brazil nuts, meditate like a champ, and run five miles a day, but it won't help you if you fall on the sidewalk and crack your skull.

Accidents are the fifth leading cause of death in America (following heart disease, cancer, stroke, and lower respiratory diseases). Home accidents alone account for 21 million medical visits a year.

Safety's not the sexiest part of the wellness industry, so accident prevention doesn't get a lot of play in the media. I'm guessing *Men's Health* wouldn't sell a lot of copies with cover lines like WALK THIS WAY: 10 HOT NEW WAYS TO AVOID SLIPPING AND FALLING. But if you want to live a long life—a crucial part of the definition of health—you've got to keep safety in mind.

The losing-my-sons incident was the catalyst for a month of safety. I've become obsessed with safety. Which is saying something, since I was pretty overprotective before.

When my first son was born, I bought the electric-outlet covers and the foam corners for the tables. As Julie will attest, I got a little carried away. I spent some time on the Internet researching whether you could buy helmets for babies. I didn't buy the helmets, but I looked. They've got such soft heads, you know? Julie mocked me hard for that one. She also mocked me for not wanting to read them *The Cat in the Hat*. But I stand by that one: Here's a boy and a girl, left alone, and what do they do? They let a smooth-talking stranger into the house. Then they try to keep the whole incident secret from their parents.

Point is, I thought I was on top of things, safetywise. It turns out I'm an accident-prevention slacker. My harmless-seeming apartment is a death trap. At least according to those who obsess about this stuff even more than I did.

I invited over Meri-K Appy, head of the nonprofit organizations Home Safety Council and Safe Kids USA. Just as my aunt Marti inspected my home for toxins Appy would scrutinize our apartment for safety violations.

When I answer the door, Appy is scanning the ceiling in the hallway.

"I was just checking to see if you have sprinklers in this building."

We don't. Strike one.

As you'd hope with a safety expert, Appy is well put together, her brown hair in a neat bob, her wardrobe a crisp blue blazer and black shirt. I was worried she'd be Nurse Ratched–severe, but she's warm and funny, prefacing some of her more hard-core suggestions with the phrase "okay, nerd alert here."

She's taken aback by how blasé we are as a society about safety. So many of us view fire alarms as a slightly less annoying version of Muzak, background noise we can freely ignore. She was recently having dinner at a Chinese restaurant when a fire alarm started honking, and everyone but her family kept happily eating their wonton soups. She couldn't resist scolding one of the alarm-flouting families on the way out.

"My feeling is that there are so many horrible, terrible ways to die that you can't do anything about. So why wouldn't you do something about the ones you can prevent?"

We start in the kitchen. This room is packed with violations. The knives are too accessible. The oven mitts are too close to the stove.

We have a smoke alarm, which is a good start. But in the kitchen? Sometimes people disable kitchen smoke alarms because they go off during cooking.

I swear I haven't. But I'm not off the hook: The smoke alarm is too old (ten years is the maximum). I need to change the batteries every year. And to be safe, I should sync this smoke alarm with the others in the house.

"Also, you should take a light vacuum and get the dust out of the smoke alarm once a month," she says. Too much dust desensitizes them.

Oh, and look into getting those sprinklers.

"I'm feeling overwhelmed," I say.

"I know it's a lot. But I'm giving you everything, and then you can do the most important."

Even Appy—the queen of safety herself—can't do it all. She admits she cooks on her stove's front burners, even though back ones are ideal from a safety perspective.

Among our many violations: A pail left in the hallway is a tripping hazard.

Our tub has no slip-resistant decals or grab bars.

Appliances are still plugged in even when not in use.

There's a glass bowl up on a top shelf.

One saving grace: Our hot water isn't that hot, far below the 110-degree danger mark. Appy says accidental scaldings are the most underestimated home hazard, responsible for more than one hundred thousand injuries a year.

She notes the candles on our dining room table. I might want to consider flameless, electric candles.

"I use them myself," she says. "There's even one with a very subtle vanilla scent."

I check to make sure Julie's not listening, since I know this would be an eye roller.

"Sometimes I worry about Hanukkah candles," I say. "Especially if we have to leave the room and they're still burning."

She nods, understandingly. She tells me she has a colleague who worked with Orthodox Jews. And he recommended putting ritual candles in the sink if they are left to burn overnight.

"And what about birthday candles?" I ask.

"I'm torn," she admits. "Because I love birthdays. But children close to an open flame? What are we teaching our kids with that? You might want to have the kids blow from far away. Some of my friends in fire safety don't have candles on the cake. They have other things, like flowers."

Julie returns and I can start speaking in a normal voice again.

"So how'd we do?" I ask.

"You didn't do too badly," she says. "I definitely give you a B or B-minus. Luckily, your kids are a little older. Otherwise, you'd get a C-minus."

The Helmet Experiment

After Appy leaves, I decide my final miniproject will be the Week of Maximum Safety.

I want to get us up to an A-plus apartment. The next morning, I spend an hour on the Internet browsing new smoke alarms and flameless candles. (I decide against the one with fake molten wax dripping down the side. It's trying too hard.) I take all the glass bowls down from the shelves. I get foot-shaped slip-resistant decals.

I also decide that to be truly, totally safe, I should investigate the idea for which Julie once ridiculed me: the helmet. Not just a helmet for biking or riding go-karts, but a helmet for walking around the city.

Strange as it sounds, I'm not the only one who has considered walking helmets. Over in Denmark in 2009, they launched a campaign that promotes helmets for pedestrians.

The Danish Road Safety Council printed posters featuring stick figures in various situations—shopping, taking the escalator, throwing out trash—all adorned with multicolored helmets. The slogan reads: "A walking helmet is a good helmet. Traffic safety isn't just for cyclists. The pedestrians of Denmark actually have a higher risk of head injury."

This was not a prank or an *Onion* story. I checked.

And what about car helmets? I'm not talking about helmets for NASCAR drivers, but helmets for your average taxi rider or suburban commuter in a Honda. Again, there have been sporadic attempts to get those in the mainstream, to little effect.

So as an experiment, I've been wearing my blue bike helmet as I run my errands. It's not so bad. I'm not getting as many quizzical stares as I predicted; passersby no doubt assume my bike or moped is locked up nearby. And there is a feeling of security. Especially when I run under New York's omnipresent scaffolding, which I've always feared.

I tried it out in the apartment as well. Tonight, I wore it while bringing the boys their plates of pasta. Julie refused to comment, but Lucas admired it so much he ran and put on his bike helmet. His has a pirate on it and thus upstaged my plain Jane helmet.

After a couple of days, I retire my walking helmet. Partly because I can't fit both my noise-canceling earphones and my helmet on my head. I had to choose.

Now, helmets for walking and driving are about as likely to take hold as capri pants for men (a very brief fashion trend I once wrote about at *Esquire*). It's just never going to happen, even in Denmark. Libertarians would go bonkers. Walking helmets are just too dorky, even for me.

But step back for a minute. Pretend you're from Mars. From a coldly rational point of view, pedestrian helmets aren't a crazy idea. As *Freakonomics* points out, on a per-mile basis, more people die from drunk walking than drunk driving. Pedestrian accidents in general kill more than twenty-five thousand people a year.

The reason I even brought up helmets is to illustrate an important point: The way we think about danger is illogical. We cannot do risk assessment to save our life. As Richard Thaler—a professor at the University of Chicago and one of the founders of the field of behavioral economics—told me, "People are terrible at knowing what is really dangerous and what isn't." We focus on the wrong dangers, the ones that get the splashy headlines, not the ones that are common or abstract.

Lisa Belkin wrote a provocative article about this topic in the *New York Times*. As she points out, the five things that cause the most injuries to children eighteen and under are car accidents, homicide (usually by someone they know), child abuse, suicide, and drowning. And the top-five things that parents are most concerned about, according to the Mayo Clinic research: kidnapping, school snipers, terrorists dangerous strangers, and drugs.

Belkin points out that we drive to the store to get "organic veggies (there is no actual data proving that organic foods increase longevity) and then check our email at the next red light (2,600 traffic deaths a year are caused by drivers using cell phones, according to a Harvard study)."

Even ten years after 9/11, I'm still jittery about taking the subway. I'm afraid some lunatic is going to blow up the C-line. So often I'll either walk or take a cab instead. Which makes no logical sense. The chance of getting hurt in a taxi accident is much higher than that of a subway bombing.

So what's a semirational person to do? I've drawn up some rules of thumb. Worry about cars, not planes. Worry about fire, not abductions. Exercise, but not so much that it interferes with spending time with your family.

And maybe, just maybe, buy a helmet.

Chapter 27

The Finish Line

I GET A WEIRD JOLT every time I log onto Skype nowadays. The address book pops up, and there, on the front page, is "Grandpa Ted." Even odder, his number has a green circle next to it, meaning that he's somehow logged in, as if they have Wi-Fi in the afterlife.

I always think of clicking on it, but decide it'd be too depressing when he never picks up.

I'm noticing these cues more and more, not just on my computer, and not just for my grandfather. As I get older, the city is filling up with morbid little landmarks of dead friends and family.

I'll walk by Nick & Toni's, an Italian joint, and think about how I ate ravioli there with an ex-girlfriend fifteen years ago. She suffered from depression and committed suicide last year in her "Obama mama" T-shirt.

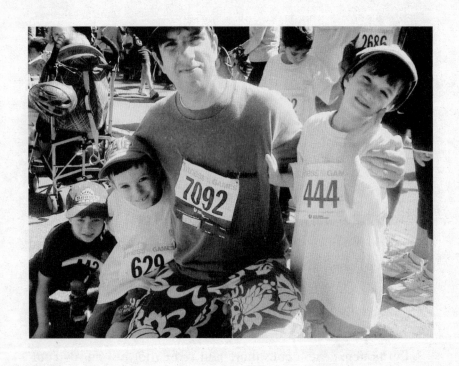

There on the corner, that's the deli where I chatted with Bob, the tech guy at *Esquire,* who died of a heart attack at fifty-one. I could do a macabre walking tour of Manhattan.

Today, I'm taking a trip into the center of it, my grandfather's old apartment on Sixty-first Street. All the grandkids are encouraged to stop by to see if there's a keepsake they want before it's all sold or stored or given away.

My mother unlocks the door of 11-F, and I smell the familiar Grandpa odor: a mix of mustiness and Johnson's baby powder. He used to pour it into his shoes every day like it was milk in cereal.

In some ways it looks like he just went out for a roast beef sandwich. The black rectangular magnifying glass he used to read with, it's lying on the living room table. The plastic chess set with see-through cubic pieces is all set up, ready for him to make an opening gambit. His Dell computer with the huge keyboard is waiting for him to start tapping out e-mails.

As we walk to the bedroom, I step on a plastic chicken drumstick that one of his great-grandkids left under the kitchen table.

In the bedroom, large cardboard boxes cover the bed. One of his daughters had labeled each box with a black Sharpie: "Books 1," "Books 2," "Photos 1," and so on. Occasionally the label has some charming editorializing, like the box that said "New York: The City That He Loved," filled with a biography of city planner Robert Moses and an award from the Urban League.

I'd come in search of one item: the suit my grandfather had worn to Julie's and my wedding. It was no ordinary suit. It was red-and-white gingham jacket and pants, and it was bold and awesome and reminded me of something Dan Aykroyd and Steve Martin's Czech brothers would have in their closet. I don't know if I'd ever have the courage to wear it in public, but I liked the idea of it in my apartment. It would be a checkerboard-patterned reminder of a life lived fully.

I swing open the closet door. There's lots of eye-squintingly bright clothes, but no sign of the suit.

"I think it was so worn out that somebody threw it away," said my mom apologetically.

"What about this?" She pulled a hanger out with a blue-and-red flower-print shirt. It's no gingham suit, but it'll suffice.

There are dozens of things left on my healthy to-do list. I haven't joined a chorus (which has been linked to reduced heart disease). I haven't eaten Japanese daikon radish or geranium extract, which is supposedly anti-inflammatory, antiviral, antibacterial, anti-everything-bad-in-the-world. I haven't returned to the Sleep Clinic for my follow-up CPAP exam.

And the body parts. What about the spleen? And the liver? And the esophagus? I haven't devoted a month to any of those.

But in the name of mental health, I have to put an end to full-time, nonstop healthy living. I promised my sons. They've been waiting patiently for two years to share cupcakes with me during birthday parties.

Am I the healthiest man alive? I'm certainly a lot healthier than I was two years ago. I went for my final exam at EHE and found out I'd lost another half pound, ending at 156.5 (total weight loss: 16 pounds). I'd gone down two belt sizes. Dr. Harry Fisch told me that my lipid panel numbers "are so good, they'll give you a heart attack" (HDL: 48, LDL: 62). I increased my VO_2 max—a lung-capacity measurement that is a good predictor of future health—by 37 percent from the start of the year. I have a visible chest.

I've hopefully boosted my longevity, despite my stubborn

refusal to move to Okinawa or Sardinia. I'll let you know in a few decades.

But the healthiest in the world? Who knows. Probably not. For one thing, I've been so busy with food and exercise, my life has teetered out of balance. I've skipped movie nights with my wife and missed pre-K presentations.

Dr. Bratman would say I've contracted a bit of orthorexia. Lately, I've been avoiding most fruits, except the bitterest one, grapefruit, afraid they are too highly glycemic.

So that's it: My days of full-throttle healthy living are over. Instead, I'll be switching to a healthier approach to health.

I'll incorporate much of what I learned.

I'll chew more. I'll walk more, and hum and pet dogs. I'll wear my noise-canceling earphones. I'll stop to smell the almonds. I'll write e-mails on my treadmill and run my errands. I'll reframe life's horrible situations and outsource my worries.

I'll floss my teeth and breathe from my stomach. I'll eat my Swiss chard and quinoa. I'll drink ice water, meditate, and give abundant thanks.

I'll try to stay married and have not-too-infrequent sex. When I exercise, I'll do High-Intensity Interval Training, alternating between sprinting and walking every minute. I'll avoid blue light before bedtime.

I'll follow fitness expert Oscar Wilde's advice: Be moderate in all things, including moderation. There's room for immoderation. Celebratory feasts can be healthy, and the occasional triathlon as well.

And I will try to have more days like June 19, the final day of my project, when Julie and I shlep the boys to Brooklyn to see a minor league baseball game featuring our local team, the Cyclones. I've walked 8,304 steps so far, many of them to get to the stadium. I'm in the open air, breathing in those phytoncides. I'm getting just a little sun exposure for my vitamin D. I'm watching baseball, which may lower blood pressure.

I've done some aerobic activity, including tossing a ball in a booth near the stadium. A radar gun tells you how fast you pitched.

The whole family tried it out. The radar malfunctioned when Zane lobbed his ball, and registered that he threw at ninety-four miles per hour. "Get that kid a contract with the Mets!" said the guy running the booth.

And right now I'm walking back to our seats, holding the little hand of my pitching prodigy, his touch suppressing my level of the stress hormone cortisol. Zane's hand is sticky, since he's currently at work on his one permitted treat for the day, a stick of blue cotton candy.

"Do you want a taste, Daddy?" he asks. He holds it aloft for me to see, a bright Q-tip of spun sugar.

I hesitate. Yes. I guess I do. Just a taste.

Guerrilla Exercise

How to turn the world into your gym

Six Tips for Normal People

1. Resist the siren song of the People Mover at airports.
2. Squat down to the level of kids when you talk to them.
3. Park in the farthest corner of the parking lot.
4. Embrace stairs, avoid elevators.
5. Fidget. Or, as scientists call it, engage in Incidental Physical Activity. Even tapping your leg can help cardiovascular fitness.
6. If you are walking in New York, cross the street by walking through the subway station, forcing you to go down and up the stairs (bonus: no waiting for red lights).

Seven Tips for the Obsessed

1. Run errands. As in run them. If you're running to any work appointments, I recommend keeping a stick of deodorant and a new shirt in your bag.

2. Have meetings like you're a character in *The West Wing*, walking and talking quickly through the office corridors.
3. Have lunch while squatting.
4. Adjust the TV by actually getting up and pressing buttons on the console.
5. Wear a weight vest all day (be prepared for suicide-bomber jokes).
6. Push the stroller and/or grocery shopping cart with the brakes on.
7. Use your children as barbells.

Appendix B

How to Eat Less

The art and science of portion control

Four Tips for Regular People

1. Get small plates. I use my sons' Nemo and Dinosaur plates.
2. Practice Chewdaism. Hard-core chewers recommend as many as fifty chews per mouthful. I strive for fifteen or twenty.
3. Turn off the TV. Studies show that we eat up to 71 percent more when we're watching TV.
4. Put the fork down in between bites

Six Tips for the Obsessed

1. Bring your own tiny fork wherever you go. Or better yet, chopsticks.
2. Repackage your pantry food (e.g., cookies, dried fruit, candy) into small Ziploc bags, so a portion is barely larger than the dime bags that pot dealers used back in the innocent eighties.

3. Write a hundred-dollar check to the KKK. Or any other equally noxious group. Then make a deal with yourself or your friend: If you eat another Ho Ho, you will have to send that check off.

4. Look at yourself. Research shows we eat less when we eat in front of a mirror.

5. Respect your elder. Digitally age a photo of yourself (you can try HourFace.com). Keep it in your wallet so that your remember to eat for your future self.

6. Eat an apple, a bowl of soup with cayenne pepper, two glasses of water, and a handful of nuts. They have all been shown to suppress the appetite. Some more details below, starting with the one I found most effective, and ending with the one I found least effective.

- Apple: A Penn State study showed that those who ate an apple fifteen minutes before lunch consumed 187 fewer calories than those who had applesauce.
- Nuts: Or beans. Or pretty much any protein makes you feel full longer than carbs. Which is why I force eggs on my kids in the morning.
- Water: A Virginia Tech study found that drinking two eight-ounce glasses of water before a meal helped obese people lose weight.
- Cayenne pepper: Spicy foods might help us lose weight, partly by curbing our urge for sugary, salty and fatty foods. A Perdue University study showed cayenne pepper lowered appetite.
- Soup: Another Penn State study recommended a small bowl of vegetable soup before the meal. The soup eaters consumed 134 fewer calories.

Five Tips on Treadmill Desks

by Joe Stirt, M.D., anesthesiologist, blogger, and treadmill-desk pioneer

1. Any working treadmill will do to get started—don't use cost as an excuse. Go to Craigslist and find one for a hundred dollars or less. Sometimes people will give you theirs free if you ask, just to get rid of it. Make sure you turn it on and walk on it before you pay for it. If it can handle 2 mph without sparking or smoking, you're money.

2. Don't be fooled by websites advertising treadmill desks for hundreds or thousands of dollars. You have most of what you need in your home and shouldn't spend more than a hundred dollars (apart from the treadmill) to get a working setup that you can tweak and modify as you go along.

3. The basic setup requires only a stack of crates, boxes or furniture in front of your treadmill stable enough to support a computer

screen and/or TV. Make the stack tall enough that the center of the screen is around eye level as you walk on the treadmill. If you're forced to look down all the time, your neck and eyes will get tired and you'll quit.

4. Now you'll want to lay a board across the treadmill handles for your keyboard. Use books atop the board to elevate the keyboard to where it's comfortable to type on. The mouse or track pad goes on either side of the keyboard.

5. Start at 0.7 mph. Yes, it's absurdly slow. But you need to get used to a whole new way of working. Gradually increase your time on the treadmill, and increase your speed in 0.1mph increments weekly to where you can work comfortably. I've been at 2.0 mph for years now, averaging three hours a day.

Within one to two weeks you will start really liking your treadmill work space and likely realize you are feeling better and doing better work than when you were a desk slug. It only gets better. Not to mention that you'll sleep better and lose weight if you stay with it. If you want more specialized tips or advice, e-mail me: bookofjoe@gmail.com.

My Five Foolproof (for Me, at Least) Methods of Stress Reduction

1. *Self-massage.* The G-rated kind. I rub my shoulders, neck, and arms daily.

2. *Outsource your worry.* Find someone to trade worries with you. Or you can try GetFriday.com, an outsourcing firm that will do almost anything legal.

3. *Meditate.* My trick: I focus on the gently pulsating light on a Mac-Book in sleep mode, and try to breathe in sync with it. I'm sure Buddhist monks do the same.

4. *Get a dog or cat.* A State University of New York–Buffalo study found that having pets present lowered stress during stressful tasks such as doing hard math problems or submerging the hand in ice water. Thankfully, my family and I are the occasional foster

parents to Daisy, a very cute and drooly basset hound owned by our friends Candice and Ben.

5. *Put the serenity prayer to work.* I've long known the prayer (God, grant me the serenity to accept the things I cannot change/Courage to change the things I can/And wisdom to know the difference). But this year, at the suggestion of several stress books, I wrote down all of my worries, and sorted them into Category A (things I can control) and Category B (things out of my control). My Category-B list was an astoundingly long one, ranging from fear of the super-volcano hiding underneath the surface of Wyoming, which may explode any day now and plunge planet Earth into an era of darkness, to the worry that my sons won't find their soul mates, to the concern that the super-volcano might kill my sons' soulmates.

Appendix 00 TK

More Appendices TK

Author's Note

All the events in this book are true. Some of the sequences have been rearranged, and, in certain cases, the names and identifying details have been changed.

This book is for informational and entertainment purposes. It's not a medical textbook. I have a B.A. after my name, not an M.D. Talk to a doctor before following any health tips in this book. And consult your spouse before moving to Okinawa.

Acknowledgments

Index

About the Author

A.J. JACOBS is the author of three *New York Times* bestsellers, including *The Know-It-All: One Man's Humble Quest to Become the Smartest Person in the World*, *The Year of Living Biblically: One Man's Humble Quest to Follow the Bible as Literally As Possible*, and *My Life as an Experiment*. He is the editor at large at *Esquire* magazine. He has also written for the *New York Times*, *The Washington Post*, and *Entertainment Weekly*. He lives in New York City. You can visit his website at ajjacobs.com.